IMAGE-GUIDED
PAIN MANAGEMENT

D1528261

IMAGE-GUIDED PAIN MANAGEMENT

Editor

P. Sebastian Thomas, M.D.
Vice Chairman
Professor of Anesthesiology
Director, Pain Treatment Service
Department of Anesthesiology
SUNY Health Science Center
Syracuse, New York

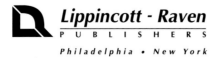

Lippincott - Raven
P U B L I S H E R S
Philadelphia • New York

Tenn. Tech. Univ. Library
Cookeville, TN 38505

Acquisitions Editor: Craig Percy
Developmental Editor: Anne Snyder
Manufacturing Manager: Dennis Teston
Production Manager: Larry Bernstein
Production Editor: Loretta Cummings
Cover Designer: Ede Driekers
Indexer: Elizabeth Babcock-Atkinson
Compositor: Lippincott-Raven Electronic Production
Printer: Kingsport Press

© 1997 by Lippincott-Raven Publishers. All rights reserved. This book is protected by copyright. No part of it may be reproduced, stored in a retrieval system, or transmitted, in any form or by any means—electronic, mechanical, photocopy, recording, or otherwise—without the prior written consent of the publisher, except for brief quotations embodied in critical articles and reviews. For information write **Lippincott-Raven Publishers, 227 East Washington Square, Philadelphia, PA 19106-3780.**

Materials appearing in this book prepared by individuals as part of their official duties as U.S. Government employees are not covered by the above-mentioned copyright.

Printed in the United States of America

9 8 7 6 5 4 3 2 1

Library of Congress Cataloging-in-Publication Data

Image-guided pain management / editor, P. Sebastian Thomas.
    p. cm.
Includes bibliographical references and index.
ISBN 0-397-51743-2
1. Pain—Treatment. 2. Imagery (Psychology)—Therapeutic use.
3. Visualization—Therapeutic use. I. Thomas, P. Sebastian
    [DNLM: 1. Pain—therapy. 2. Nerve Block. 3. Diagnostic Imaging.
WL 704 I31 1997]
RB127.I43 1997
616'.0472–dc20
DNLM/DLC
For Library of Congress

Care has been taken to confirm the accuracy of the information presented and to describe generally accepted practices. However, the authors, editors, and publisher are not responsible for errors or omissions or for any consequences from application of the information in this book and make no warranty, express or implied, with respect to the contents of the publication.

The authors, editors, and publisher have exerted every effort to ensure that drug selection and dosage set forth in this text are in accordance with current recommendations and practice at the time of publication. However, in view of ongoing research, changes in government regulations, and the constant flow of information relating to drug therapy and drug reactions, the reader is urged to check the package insert for each drug for any change in indications and dosage and for added warnings and precautions. This is particularly important when the recommended agent is a new or infrequently employed drug.

Some drugs and medical devices presented in this publication have Food and Drug Administration (FDA) clearance for limited use in restricted research settings. It is the responsibility of the health care provider to ascertain the FDA status of each drug or device planned for use in their clinical practice.

To my best friend and wife, Alice

Contents

Contributing Authors

Christi Barber, R.N., N.P.   *Department of Anesthesiology, SUNY Health Science Center at Syracuse, 750 East Adams Street, Syracuse, New York 13210*

Scott C. Buckingham, M.D.   *Assistant Professor, Interventional Radiologist, Department of Radiology, SUNY Health Science Center at Syracuse, 750 East Adams Street, Syracuse, New York 13210*

John J. Cambareri, M.D.   *Assistant Professor, Department of Anesthesiology, SUNY Health Science Center at Syracuse, 750 East Adams Street, Syracuse, New York 13210*

Paramjit S. Chopra, M.D.   *Assistant Professor of Radiology, Chief, Cardiovascular and Interventional Radiology, SUNY Health Science Center at Syracuse, 750 East Adams Street, Syracuse, New York 13210*

David G. Fellows, M.D.   *Assistant Professor, Associate Director, Pain Treatment Service, Department of Anesthesiology, SUNY Health Science Center at Syracuse, 750 East Adams Street, Syracuse, New York 13210*

Bruce E. Fredrickson, M.D.   *Professor of Orthopedic and Neurologic Surgery, Spine Center, Department of Orthopedics, SUNY Health Science Center at Syracuse, 750 East Adams Street, Syracuse, New York 13210*

Leo Hochhauser, M.D., F.R.C.P.C.   *Associate Professor, Neuroradiologist, Department of Radiology, SUNY Health Science Center at Syracuse, 750 East Adams Street, Syracuse, New York 13210*

James W. Holsapple, M.D.   *Assistant Professor, Department of Neurological Surgery, SUNY Health Science Center at Syracuse, 750 East Adams Street, Syracuse, New York 13210*

Syed I. Hosain, F.R.C.A.   *Clinical Instructor, Pain Treatment Service, Department of Anesthesiology, SUNY Health Science Center at Syracuse, 750 East Adams Street, Syracuse, New York 13210*

Thomas D. Masten, M.D.   *Assistant Professor, Department of Orthopedic Surgery, SUNY Health Science Center at Syracuse, 750 East Adams Street, Syracuse, New York 13210*

Nitin P. Shirodkar, M.D.   *Resident, Radiology Department, University of Buffalo, Medical and Dental Consortium, Buffalo, New York 14214*

Andrew M. Sopchak, M.D.   *Resident, Radiology Department, University of Buffalo, Medical and Dental Consortium, Buffalo, New York 14214*

P. Sebastian Thomas, M.D.   *Vice Chairman, Professor of Anesthesiology, Director, Pain Treatment Service, Department of Anesthesiology, SUNY Health Science Center at Syracuse, 750 East Adams Street, Syracuse, New York 13210*

Jeffrey S. Wang, M.D.   *Clinical Instructor, Pain Treatment Service, Department of Anesthesiology, SUNY Health Science Center at Syracuse, 750 East Adams Street, Syracuse, New York 13210*

Paul H. Willoughby, M.D.   *Assistant Professor, Pain Treatment Service, Department of Anesthesiology, SUNY Health Science Center at Syracuse, 750 East Adams Street, Syracuse, New York 13210*

Pramod Yadhati, M.D.   *Clinical Instructor, Pain Treatment Service, Department of Anesthesiology, SUNY Health Science Center at Syracuse, 750 East Adams Street, Syracuse, New York 13210*

Preface

Since 1981, when I finished my fellowship in pain management and began my career, the complexity of intervention procedures has increased dramatically. Although the use of X-rays
and CT scans in pain management is quite common, many pain
practitioners are still uncomfortable using and interpreting
these images. As the popularity of pain fellowships continues
to grow, young physicians who wish to obtain optimum train-
ing in pain management should have a good understanding of
all image-guided procedures.

Obviously, not all nerve blocks need to be done under fluoroscopic guidance. A good majority of the procedures performed for pain management have definite anatomical landmarks and objective tests for accurate localization. These
include eliciting paresthesias and using large volumes of local
anesthetic agents to obtain sensory blockades.

In this book, I have tried to emphasize the most complex and
difficult procedures used in pain management. The first two
chapters are intended to familiarize readers with the use of X-
rays, CT scans, and radio-opaque dyes. Most of the subsequent
chapters deal with the specifics of the performance of blocks,
and only briefly discuss the indications and complications. I
hope that pain practitioners will find this book useful in their
daily practice.

P. Sebastian Thomas, M.D.

Acknowledgments

I would like to extend my appreciation to the Department of Anesthesiology at SUNY Health Science Center at Syracuse, New York, for its help and support in making this endeavor successful. I wish to express my fondest regards and appreciation to Howard L. Zauder, M.D., who gave me the opportunity to do what I wanted to do and helped me to be what I am today.

In particular, I wish to thank Mary Corbett and Mary Jo DiNuzzo for their dedicated work in preparing and collating the manuscripts, and Christi Barber, R.N., N.P. for the many hours she spent in putting it all together. This book could not have been completed without their hard work and dedication.

IMAGE-GUIDED
PAIN MANAGEMENT

IMAGE-GUIDED PAIN MANAGEMENT
edited by P. S. Thomas.
Lippincott–Raven Publishers, Philadelphia © 1997

1

Image-Guided Needle Localization: Fluoroscopy and Computed Tomography Scan

Scott C. Buckingham and Leo Hochhauser

*Department of Radiology, SUNY Health Science Center at Syracuse,
Syracuse, New York 13210*

The 100th anniversary of the discovery of the x-ray was marked in 1995. The original x-ray studies were simply transmission exposures on film. Since that time x-ray technology has augmented almost all medical specialties and its use has increased dramatically. This is not only reflected in the dramatic increase in the volume of standard film screen studies but also, as technology progressed, by the addition of newer modalities such as fluoroscopy and computed tomography (CT). These techniques have evolved tremendously since their introduction with considerably improved image quality, diminished imaging time, and reduced patient radiation dose.

As with film screen studies, fluoroscopy and CT use transmitted x-rays to create imaging information. However, they use different and more complex means of processing and displaying the data acquired. Modern CT and fluoroscopy offer high resolution images and rapid display of information thus providing real-time imaging guidance for invasive procedures.

FLUOROSCOPIC GUIDANCE

Fluoroscopically generated images begin with the transmission of a beam of x-rays through a subject. The beam originates from a generator tube and can be approximated as beginning from a point source. It spreads slightly as it travels through the subject and reaches the detector leading to some geometric magnification (Fig. 1).

The detector and display systems for fluoroscopy have improved tremendously over the years. Early systems relied on transmitted x-rays striking a fluorescent screen which was viewed directly. The image was so dim that viewing required prior acclimation to dim light conditions. Modern systems use image intensification to multiply the small electrical signal produced by the transmitted x-rays to many thousands of times its original strength. Display is via the closed circuit TV which allows further manipulation of image display. These developments allow convenient use of fluoroscopy to guide invasive procedures in workable lighting conditions with immediate display of imaging information.

Guiding needle placement under fluoroscopy requires the understanding of basic imaging principals. Foremost is the understanding that the three dimensions of the subject are rep-

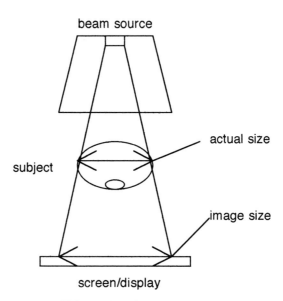

FIG. 1. Magnification of beam.

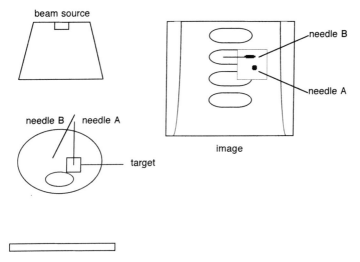

FIG. 2. Straight shot approach.

resented as two dimensions on the display monitor screen. The missing depth dimension must be inferred. Although this is best achieved by viewing the subject at a 90° angle to the first imaging plane, this is only feasible if the x-ray tube can be rotated along an arc (C-arm) or if a second tube is available preferably mounted at a right angle to the other.

Depth can be assessed in a variety of ways including relationship to bony landmarks, change in appearance and orientation of the needle on various oblique views, and position and orientation of the needle relative to the patient.

A simple method of guiding a needle in the correct direction is to use the "down the barrel" or straight shot approach (Fig. 2). Once an appropriate site on the skin surface is selected for needle entry, an oblique view is obtained with the x-ray beam directly in line with the desired needle path. The needle will appear as a dot over the target and increasing deviation from the path will be reflected on the display image by seeing an increasing length of the needle shaft.

Depth to the target can be determined at any point during needle advancement by temporarily rotating to a new obliquity perpendicular to the first viewing plane. A biplane fluoroscopic system can provide a significant time advantage in this situation by allowing immediate or simultaneous assessment of needle position from the second imaging system (Fig. 3). If the target is a solid bony structure, an experienced operator will often not require any depth assessment and can advance in the correct direction until encountering the expected resistance of the target.

In some circumstances it may not be possible or desirable to use a straight shot approach for needle placement. In such cases, a variety of other methods to ensure correct position must be used. Comparison of oblique views is often useful in this situation. This approach is based on geometric principals of object position and beam direction. In simplest terms, as the x-ray beam is rotated through an arc of oblique views, anterior objects move in the opposite direction of posterior objects. A needle tip which appears to be directly over the target on a frontal view can be assessed in this manner to determine if correctly positioned or actually anterior or posterior to the desired location (Fig. 4).

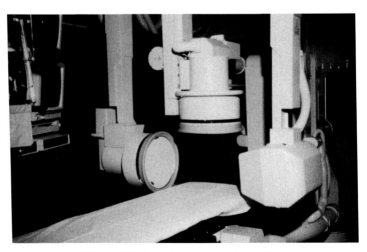

FIG. 3. Bi-plane fluoroscopic laboratory.

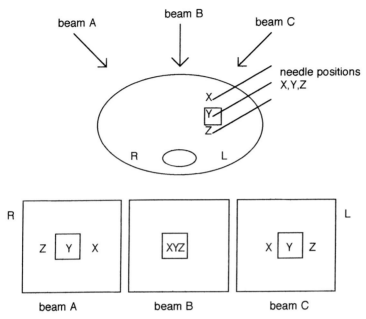

FIG. 4. Anterior and posterior positioning.

Even when one knows exactly where the needle is situated and where one would like it to end up, directing the needle to the target may present some difficulty at times. Whereas experience is the best teacher in handling each case, some tricks may be used to help in directing a needle pass.

Needles with symmetric tips tend to track straighter than those with asymmetric tips. If you are using a beveled needle, know the direction of the bevel. This is often marked by a notch on the needle hub. Plan ahead for some slight deviation in needle track with a beveled tip. Redirecting the angle of the bevel when only partway advanced can help to steer back onto course.

Larger gauge and stiffer needles generally track straighter. This must be balanced with the additional patient discomfort and risk of a larger needle. A helpful compromise is coaxial technique. A larger guiding needle can be placed through superficial or fascial layers. Through this needle a smaller gauge needle can then be advanced to the target directed by the stiffer outer guiding needle. If the guiding needle is slightly off course it can often still be used by putting a slight bend into the tip of the inner needle allowing it to be redirected as it passes out the end of the guiding catheter. It is helpful to know the relationship of the bend to the bevel marker on the needle hub as the direction can not otherwise be identified while the inner needle is within the guiding needle.

Another means of redirecting a needle during passage is to induce a deflecting curve. This can be done by pushing or pulling the superficial tissues after the needle is partially placed to angle it in the desired direction. It may also be done by placing a finger or a thumb against the needle at the skin entry site and inducing a bow in the needle with the other hand. The needle can then be advanced along the course of the resulting curve. This is most successful with needles of moderate stiffness.

Advantages of fluoroscopic guidance include ready availability, low cost, and high spatial resolution. In most cases, imaging in a variety of planes is easily accomplished. Disadvantages include the inherent lack of soft tissue contrast (inability to distinguish different soft tissue structures, i.e., muscle from the aorta) and the exposure of individuals performing the procedure as well as the patient to ionizing radiation.

COMPUTED TOMOGRAPHIC GUIDANCE

CT has developed from relatively low spatial resolution systems which required minutes to hours to produce an image into current systems that produce high resolution images in seconds. It is the rapid production of images with outstanding contrast resolution and good spatial resolution which make CT the optimal choice for guiding invasive procedures in certain circumstances.

CT scanners (Fig. 5) generate a circumferential or helical projection of x-rays back through the patient to a detection system on the opposite side. This information is collected and used to calculate a map of attenuation values of each point

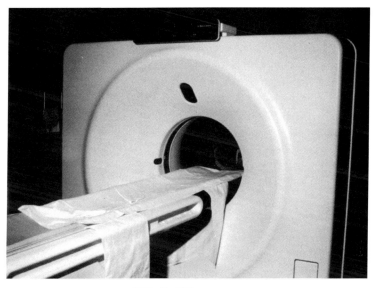

FIG. 5. CT scanner.

within the scanned area of the subject. Attenuation can be equated with density for the purpose of this discussion. The scanned area is essentially a slice, the thickness of which can be varied by the CT operator. Within this slice each coordinate location denotes a 3D volume element or voxel (the volume equivalent of a 2D picture element or pixel). The voxel size is defined by the pixel dimensions in the plane of the slice—which also determines spatial resolution—and the slice thickness. The average attenuation within this volume is displayed on the image as a grayscale pixel. The grayscale value corresponding to given densities can be varied by the operator to optimize definition of the tissues of interest.

Targeting of needle placement under CT facilitates a safer and more accurate result in many circumstances where fluoroscopy would not provide satisfactory identification of the target or adjacent structures which may have to be avoided. On the other hand, it does not allow real-time imaging of the advancement of the needle.

Under optimal circumstances for CT guidance the target and an acceptable entry site are visualized on the same scan slice with a straight path between them avoiding any structures that should not be crossed with the needle. Obviously, each case is different with regard to risks and benefits of passing a needle though such areas as liver, lung, bowel etc., and must be determined by the clinician and patient.

With an acceptable approach defined by the CT scan and localized by some radiopaque marking on the skin surface, the entry site can be prepped and a small 25-gauge needle placed at the estimated proper angulation into the subcutaneous tissues. A repeat scan is useful to confirm location and angle prior to placing the procedure needle. The marking needle is often left in place initially as a guide. The procedure needle is then advanced stepwise with intermittent repeat images to confirm proper needle course and distance to the target. The number of images required will depend on the experience of the person performing the procedure and the difficulty of the particular case. The technologist performing the scan can supply exact depth, distance, and angle measurements during the procedure.

There are fewer ways to safely redirect a needle pass under CT given the lack of real-time imaging. The coaxial technique provides the same advantages and is equally useful. Placing a bend in the inner needle tip of a coaxial system (as just described) to correct for slight errors in guiding needle position is particularly helpful under CT. Inducing bowing or curve in the needle can be done but requires some experience in estimating the results of the maneuver because it can not be visualized during needle advancement. Obviously, a straight shot approach or use of different obliquities is not applicable to CT guidance.

In many cases, it is possible to obtain a slightly different targeting plane by angling the gantry of the CT scanner. This may provide a direct approach to the target that was not present with the gantry in neutral position. The needle can then be passed while remaining in the scanning slice. The correct obliquity for remaining within the slice can be estimated by observing the angle of the gantry relative to the patient and needle.

In some cases, it is necessary to pass the needle through a course that can only be visualized on multiple adjacent slices. In this case, one must obtain enough slices to ensure that the needle tip itself is visualized rather than a portion of the needle.

The principle of volume averaging must also be kept in mind. Because any pixel actually represents a volume, it will reflect the contents of that volume. This is particularly relevant with small targets or narrow paths of safe passage. A 1 ml thick needle can be anywhere within the 1-cm thick image slice it is displayed on. A target at one end of the slice and needle at the other may appear superimposed. Generally, after initial localization, thinner slices should be used if needed to accurately resolve the target from surrounding structures.

The primary advantage of CT guidance is excellent contrast resolution allowing better delineation of soft tissue structures. The patient still is exposed to ionizing radiation but no significant exposure occurs for those performing the procedure. Disadvantages include greater cost and lesser availability as well as the inability to visualize needle manipulations in real-time. Many procedures likely require longer to complete under CT as well.

RADIATION SAFETY

Both of these methods require patient exposure to ionizing radiation. Fluoroscopic guidance also leads to exposure of the health care worker. The goal is to optimize benefit while minimizing risk. ALARA (*As Low As Reasonably Achievable*) is a useful concept in which the physician and radiologic technologist bear primary responsibility for taking all steps possible to lower the patient dose to the lowest degree possible while safely completing the procedure. This includes, among other things, coning the fluoroscopic image in to the smallest area possible, shielding portions of the patient that may be exposed to scatter outside the imaging area, limiting the fluoroscopic time to the minimum possible, and maintaining equipment in good working order. During fluoroscopic work one must also be diligent in limiting dose to health care workers. All persons should wear proper shielding. Awareness of the direction of the x-ray beam to minimize exposure to scatter can reduce worker dose. The need to limit having one's hands regularly exposed to direct fluoroscopy can not be overstated. In the past, prior to realization of the risks of x-ray exposure, malignancies in the hands of radiologists who routinely placed their hands in the imaging field were not unheard of.

For CT the dose is based on the volume studied and the number of slices. Because dose is volume weighted, a diagnostic study has nearly the same dose distributed over the area studied. However, for a procedure there are likely to be several scans made through the same area and the dose is additive. This should be kept in mind particularly if the slice includes a highly radiosensitive structure.

Far more information regarding radiation safety is available than can be covered here. The radiation safety officer or radiation physicist at an institution should be able to provide adequate information as well as specific dose values for the equipment in use at a particular site.

IMAGE-GUIDED PAIN MANAGEMENT
edited by P. S. Thomas.
Lippincott–Raven Publishers, Philadelphia © 1997

2

Contrast Media in Radiologic Imaging

Paramjit S. Chopra and Nitin P. Shirodkar

Department of Radiology, SUNY Health Science Center at Syracuse, Syracuse, New York 13210

Intravascular contrast is administered to millions of patients every year in the United States. Intravascular contrast agents are used in every aspect of radiologic imaging ranging from intravenous urography and diagnostic arteriography to ultrasound and magnetic resonance imaging (MRI).

In order to understand why contrast agents are necessary for imaging it is first essential to understand the basic principles of radiography. An x-ray beam from an x-ray source passes through the body (Fig. 1). Tissues within the body attenuate the beam (by absorbing some of the x-ray's energy) based on their physical characteristics. The residual x-ray beam then reacts with the film (or other image receptor) to produce an image in proportion to the amount of x-ray energy received by the receptor (Fig. 2).

Bone with abundant calcium and a compact structure absorbs and therefore attenuates more energy from the x-ray beam than adjacent muscle. This provides inherent natural contrast between bone and adjacent soft tissues.

When two adjacent organs, whose tissues have similar attenuation characteristics, attenuate an x-ray beam equally, they cast a similar radiographic image, making it impossible to differentiate between them (e.g., blood vessels are not visualized on a plain x-ray of any part of the body because blood vessels

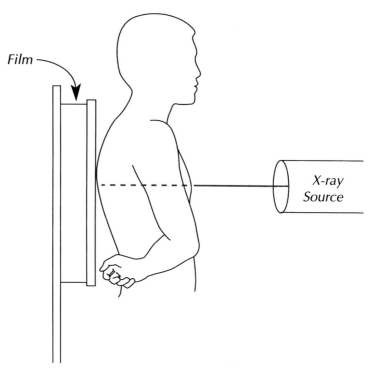

FIG. 1. Diagrammatic representation of the acquisition of a chest x-ray.

filled with blood attenuates an x-ray beam as much as the adjacent muscle and other soft tissues (Fig. 3).

In order to differentiate between two adjacent tissues with similar attenuation characteristics, it is essential to introduce a substance into the organ (blood vessel, genitourinary tract, gastrointestinal tract, subarachnoid space) (Fig. 4) to provide attenuation of x-rays.

TYPES OF CONTRAST AGENTS

Radiology has evolved from a science primarily using x-rays to other newer technologies such as ultrasound and magnetic resonance imaging (MRI). Imaging with each modality

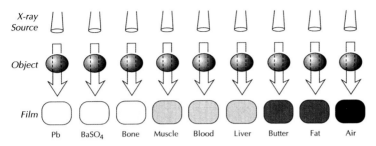

FIG. 2. Contrast obtained due to the differing attenuation of tissues and substances with the same thickness.

requires the distinction between different adjacent tissues. Various contrast agents have been developed for each of these modalities. Contrast agents can range from natural substances such as air, oxygen, and carbon dioxide gas which provide "negative" contrast. Carbon dioxide is now under investigation as an intravascular agent. These agents when inserted into the lumen of a viscera attenuate the x-ray beam less than adjoining tissue. "Positive" contrast agents are those that attenuate the x-ray beam more than the adjoining soft tissues (barium sulfate ($BaSO_4$), iodine). Iodine-based agents are used mainly in the vascular system. However, they are also used to opacify the lumen of viscera or other organ systems when a water soluble agent is needed (e.g., bile ducts—cholangiography; joint spaces—arthrography; intra-thecal spaces—myelography).

An ideal agent should be a good absorber of x-rays within the diagnostic energy range; it must be nontoxic without any adverse-associated toxicity and it should not change the physiological function of the organ where it is being used. For intravascular use, the contrast agent solution, in addition to the aforementioned criteria, must be injectable and iso-osmolar with plasma. Most intravascular agents are iodine containing compounds, in which case the iodine molecule should be on a molecule with low toxicity. These agents must pass through the pulmonary, cardiac, and peripheral capillary circulations and be stable for recirculation. Finally, they must be completely excreted from the body.

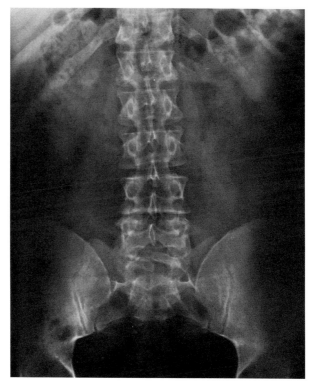

FIG. 3. Plain radiograph of the abdomen.

Iodine-Based Contrast Agents

Table 1 lists the common types of iodinated contrast agents used today. The iodinated contrast used today are water soluble compounds. They are classified into ionic and nonionic agents. Each is further classified into monomers and dimers.

Ionic Contrast Agents

The ionic contrast agents have two generalized molecular structures: (a) *ionic monomer* (monoacidic monomer), and (b) *ionic dimer* (monoacidic dimer). The ionic media dissociate in water and liberate an anion and a cation.

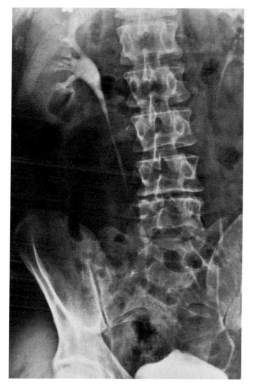

FIG. 4. Radiograph of the abdomen (25-minute film of an intravenous urogram) of the same patient as in Fig. 3. The contrast excreted by the kidneys is useful in delineating the pelvicalyceal system, the ureters and the urinary bladder without and with contrast.

Ionic Monomer

The ionic monomer is a tri-iodinated derivative of benzoic acid (Fig. 5), formulated as a salt with cations of sodium or meglumine, an organic molecule. They have a carboxyl group on position 1 of the ring. Therefore, each molecule has a valence of 1. Side groups at position 3 and 5 of the ring vary among the different compounds. The molecules have a ratio of three iodine particles for two particles in solution (ratio 1.5 molecule).

TABLE 1. *Ionic agents*

Generic name	Manufacturer
Diatrizoate	Shering, AG, Winthrop
Metrizoate	Nycomed
Iothalamate	Mallinckrodt
Iodamide	Bracco
Ioxithalamate	Guerbet
Ioglicate	Schering AG
Ioxaglate	Guerbet

These compounds are very soluble in water and have very little interaction with organic molecules. They have low molecular weights ranging between 600 and 700, and are extremely low lipid solubility. Therefore, these compounds distribute in the extra-cellular space easily and are eliminated primarily by filtration at the renal glomerular capillaries (1,2). Diatrizoate (Renografin, Hypaque-M Nycomed, Princeton, NJ) is a good example of this class of contrast agent.

Ionic Dimer (Monoacidic Dimer)

The second type of an ionic agent is the ionic dimer, also known (Fig. 6) as a monoacidic dimer. The molecule is formed by joining two ionic monomer molecules at two R side groups. The carboxyl group on one of the ionic monomers is replaced by an organic group. This leaves the dimer molecule with a

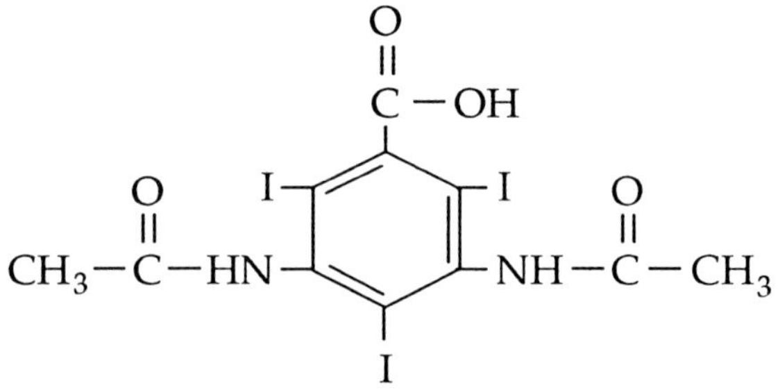

FIG. 5. Chemical structure of the ionic monomer.

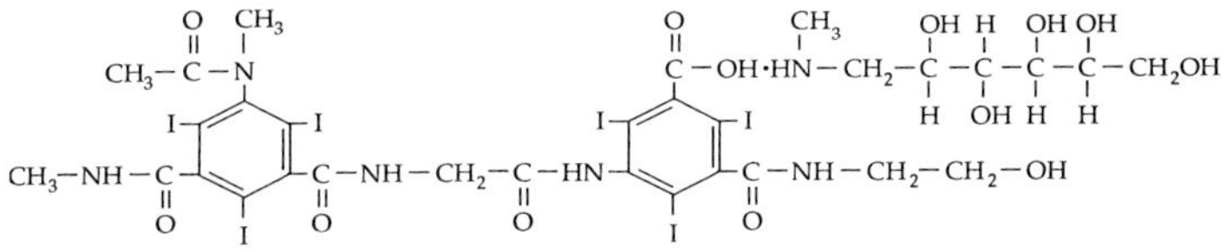

FIG. 6. Chemical structure of an ionic dimer.

valence of −1. The molecule has a ratio of six iodine atoms for two particles in solution.

The dimers, too, are very soluble in water, interact very little with organic molecules, and have an extremely low lipid solubility. Although their molecular weights are higher than the monomers (around 1200), they are still small enough to have distribution characteristics similar to ionic monomers. Ioxaglate (commercially available as Hexabrix (Mallinckrodt, Hazelwood, Mississippi), is the only commercially available dimer.

NONIONIC CONTRAST AGENTS

Nonionic contrast agents (Table 2), contrary to their ionic counterparts, do not dissociate in solution. Their osmolality is half that of ionic agents because the number of particles in solution per ioodine molecule is half that of the ionic agents. Although their molecular weights are larger than ionic agents, they too are distributed and eliminated similar to the ionic agents. The nonionic monomers used today include Iopamidol (Isovue (Bracco Diagnostic, Cranberry, NJ)), Iohexol (omnipaque (Nycomed, Princeton, New Jersey)) and Loversol (opti-

TABLE 2. *Nonionic agents*

Generic name	Manufacturer
Metrizamide	Nycomed
Iohexol	Nycomed
Iopamidol	Bracco
Iopromide	Schering AG

ray, Mallinckrodt, Hazelwood, Mississippi). Nonionic dimers include Iotrol [Schering AG] and Iodixanol.

Of all the different properties of iodinated contrast media, osmolality correlates the most with the general biological effects of contrast media. Of all the agents, nonionic dimers have the least osmolality, whereas ionic monomer have the highest osmolality.

Adverse Reactions to Contrast Media

Acute reactions can occur with all intravenous contrast agents; however, they are more common with ionic agents than with nonionic low-osmolar agents. In a review of 340,000 patients by Katayama, et al. (3), the overall incidence of reactions for ionic contrast agent was 12.66%, whereas that for nonionic contrast agents was 3.13%. However, severe reactions had an incidence of 0.22% for ionic agents and 0.04% for nonionic agents. The study also estimated that nonionic agents were six times safer than ionic contrast media.

Ionic Contrast

Most reactions to contrast media are minor and self-limited and do not have any residual effect (4). Five to eight percent of all patients receiving contrast media experience some form of reaction. Approximately 0.05% (1 in 2000) will have a reaction requiring hospitalization (need reference), and approximately 0.0025% (1 in 40,000) reactions are fatal (Palmer Australasian study).

The use of low osmolality contrast media (LOCM) has remarkably decreased the number of acute reactions. Overwhelming evidence is available documenting that the incidence of contrast reaction is significantly lower with LOCM compared to ionic media (3,5–9).

Acute reactions to contrast media (CM) may be (a) minor, (b) intermediate, or (c) severe. Minor reactions occur in approximately 5% of IV injections and include nausea, sensation of warmth, and pain. Intermediate reactions occur in 0.022% of IV injections and include severe vomiting, dyspnea, hypotension, and chest pain. Severe reactions include shock (anaphylaxis), pulmonary edema, cardiac arrhythmia, myocardial infarction, and death; they occur in approximately 0.0025% of IV injections.

Explanations for reactions to contrast media include: allergy to the iodine in the contrast agent (10), complement activation (11) in cases of the rare consumptive coagulopathy, hyperosmolality (12), and central nervous system effects (13). Several factors affect the occurrence of contrast reaction (14). Notable facts include: (a) severe reactions and death common in patients over 60; (b) cardiac disease increases the risk 4 to 5 times; (c) previous reaction increases the risk 11 times; (d) asthma increases the risk 5 times; and (e) history of allergies increases the risk 4 times.

Death (15) from severe reactions to contrast medium has occurred due to cardiac arrest, myocardial infarction, arrhythmia, respiratory arrest, and glottic edema.

Prevention of Contrast Reactions

Contrast reactions may be prevented by (a) careful screening of patients, (b) alleviating anxiety during the procedure, (c) prophylaxis with corticosteroids in the high-risk patient, and (d) use of low osmolar contrast agents. Because LOCM are exorbitantly expensive (10 to 15 times the cost of ionic contrast agents) the American College of Radiology has provided criteria for their use.

Treatment of Acute Contrast Reactions (16)

The most worrisome of reactions to contrast media is the acute anaphylactic reaction. Avoiding the reactions by identifying high-risk patients and the use of preventive measures are the most important aspects of management. Preventive measures include pre-treatment with corticosteroids and antihista-

TABLE 3. *Treatment of contrast reactions (adapted from reference contrast manual)*

Reaction	Severity	Treatment
Urticaria	Mild	observation diphenhydramine (Benadryl), 50 mg po/im/iv
	Severe	cimetidine (Tagamet), 300 mg, diluted, slow iv (pediatric: 5–10 mg/kg, diluted, slow iv) ranitidine (Zantac), 50 mg, diluted, slow iv
Bronchospasm (isolated)		Oxygen (3 L/mm) Beta-2-agonist metered dose inhaler (MDI): 2–3 deep inhalations of metaproterenol (Alupent), terbutaline (Brethaire), or albuterol (Proventil) Epinephrine (Adrenalin) Subcutaneously: 1:1000, 0.1–0.2 mL (0.1–0.2 mg); (pediatric: 0.1–0.2 mL subcutaneously) Intravenous: 1:10,000, 1 mL (0.1 mg), slow iv (pediatric: 0.01 mg/kg IV)
Anaphylactoid reaction (generalized)		Oxygen (3 L/min) fluids: normal saline Epinephrine (Adrenalin) Subcutaneously: 1:1000, 0.1–0.2 mL (0.1–0.2 mg) (pediatric: 0.1–0.2 mL) Intravenous: 1:10,000, 1 mL (0.1 mg), slowly (10 μg/min) (pediatric: 0.01 mg/kg iv) Antihistamines H1-blocker diphenhydramine, 50 mg intravenous H2-blocker cimetidine (Tagamet), 300 mg, diluted, slowly iv (pediatric: 5–10 mg/kg, diluted, slowly) ranitidine (Zantac), 50 mg, diluted, slowly iv Beta-2-agonist metered dose inhaler (MDI) (2 or 3 inhalations): metaproterenol (Alupent); terbutaline (Brethaire); albuterol (Proventil) Corticosteroids: hydrocortisone (Solu-Cortef), 0.5–1.0 g intravenous methylprednisolone (Solu-Medrol), 500 mg IV over seconds; or 2000 mg over 30 minutes

TABLE 3. *(cont'd)*

Reaction	Severity	Treatment
Hypotension	(isolated)	Oxygen (3 L/min) IV fluids (primary therapy): rapidly, normal saline Vasopressor dopamine: iv solution, 25 µg/kg/min epinephrine: iv solution, 4–8 µg/min

Vagal reaction
  (hypotension
and
bradycardia)
		Oxygen (3 L/mm)
		IV fluids: rapidly, normal saline
		Atropine: 0.8–1.0 mg iv, repeat q 3–5
		  minutes to 3 mg total (pediatric: 0.2
		  mg/kg iv; maximum 0.6 mg to 2 mg
		  total)

minics and close monitoring of the high-risk patient receiving contrast media. Once a reaction has occurred, quick recognition is vital as the anaphylactic reaction can worsen and become life threatening very rapidly.

General measures for the treatment of the acute anaphylactic reactions include (a) rapid assessment of the extent and severity of the reaction; (b) discontinuation of further administration; (c) close monitoring of vital signs, cardiac rhythm, and pulmonary function; (d) determination of the patient's medical history and current medication status; and (e) maintenance of adequate oxygenation, cardiac output, and tissue perfusion. All patients who have serious anaphylaxis should be hospitalized and monitored for at least 24 hours, because relapses may occur. Table 3 lists the treatment options for the different types of reactions to contrast media.

Contrast-Induced Nephrotoxicity

The kidneys excrete 99% of the water soluble contrast agents. Less than 1% is excreted by extra-renal routes (vicarious excretion) such as the liver, bile, small and large bowel, tears, sweat, and saliva. This vicarious excretion is seen commonly in the presence of renal failure. Administration of iodi-nated contrast media can lead to acute renal failure. The inci-dence of renal failure varies from 0–10% and has been reported to be as high as 50% (17,18). Risk factors for contrast-induced acute renal failure (17,18) include: pre-existing renal insuffi-ciency, diabetes mellitus, dehydration, cardiovascular disease, age more than 70 years, multiple myeloma, hypertension, and hyperuricemia. The etiology is due to damage to the cytoplasm of the proximal renal tubules; this is believed to be due to chemotoxicity rather than osmolality (this injury can be seen with both ionic and nonionic agents). Claims that LOCM are less nephrotoxic are still controversial (19).

CONTRAST AGENTS IN MRI

Types of Contrast Agents

The main agents used in MRI are injectable compounds approved for clinical use by the FDA. These agents produce an increase in signal intensity on T1-weighted images by enhanc-ing T1 relaxivity (for more information on the physics of MRI, the reader is referred to any standard text book on Magnetic Resonance Imaging).

These compounds include Gadopentetate Dimeglumine ((Gd-DTPA) Magnevist, Berlex Laboratories, Newark, New Jersey); Gadoteridol ((Gd-HP-DO3A) ProHance, Squibb Diag-nostics, Princeton, New Jersey); and Gadodiamide ((Gd-DTPA-BMA) Omniscan, Sanofi-Winthrop, Princeton, New Jersey). These agents are reasonably similar in terms of their enhanced properties (Figs. 7 and 8), and safety.

Other contrast agents such as super-paramagnetic iron oxide particles are under investigation for use in the hepatobiliary system. These agents induce localized susceptibility changes in tissues and produce a loss of signal on T2-weighted images.

A brief description of Gadopentetate Dimeglumine ((Gd-DTPA) Magnevist, Berlex Laboratories) is presented. The agent is a chelate formulated as a meglumine salt. It consists of a gadolinium ion and DTPA (diethyl triamine penta acetate).

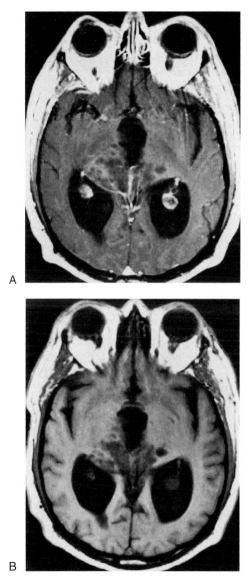

A

B

FIG. 7. MRI of the head prior to and following the injection of Gadopentetate Dimeglumine (Gd-DTPA). Note the enhancement of the choroid plexus within the lateral ventricles.

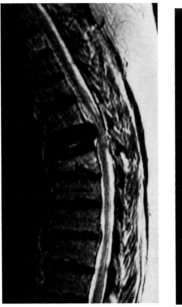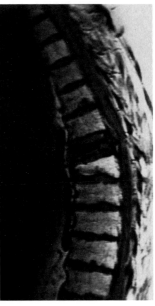

A   B

FIG. 8. MRI of the thoracic spine, prior to and following the injection of Gadopentetate Dimeglumine (Gd-DTPA). The enhanced scan better demonstrates the compression of the spinal cord by the compressed fracture of the vertebral body.

It is most commonly used for evaluation of lesions in the central nervous system (head and spine). Use in other organ systems continues to increase as experience with the agents grows. In the CNS the contrast agent helps in the detection of primary and metastatic neoplastic lesions, infection, demyelinating diseases, infarction, and arteriovenous malformations.

Contraindications

Relative contraindications to the use of Gadopentate includes hemolytic anemia (Gadopentate can cause mild transient hemolysis leading to elevation of serum iron and bilirubin), Wilson's disease, and a history of anaphylactic reactions.

Absolute (20) contraindications include pregnancy (Gado-pentate dimeglumine crosses the placenta), lactation (excreted in breast milk) and renal failure (agent excreted entirely by the kidneys). Use in children under the age of 2 years has not yet been evaluated.

Complications (21) following the use of Gadopentate are few and include minor complications such as headache, nausea and vomiting, and rash. Major complication such as a severe anaphylactic reaction is possible and has been reported. The treatment of an anaphylactic reaction to Gadopentate is the same as that for reactions occurring following the use of iodi-nated contrast media.

REFERENCES

1. Dean PB, Kivisaari L, Konmano M. The diagnostic potential of contrast enhancement pharmacokinetics. *Invest Radiol* 1978;13:533–540.
2. Donaldson ML. Comparison of renal clearance of insulin and radioactive diatrizoate as measures of glomerular filtration rate in man. *Clin Sci* 1968;35:513–524.
3. Katayama H, Yamaguchi K, Takashima T, Seez P, Matsuura K. [Adverse reactions to ionic and non-ionic contrast media: a report from the Japan-ese Committee on the safety of contrast media]. *Radiology* 1990; 175:621–628.
4. Barnhard HJ, White FA. The emergency treatment of reactions to con-trast media. Abrams Angiography. *Vascular and Interventional Radiol-ogy, 3rd ed.* 1983;1:79–94.
5. Palmer. The RACR survey of intravenous contrast media reactions [Final Report]. *Australas Radiol* 1988;32:426–428.
6. Schrott KM, Behrends B, et al. Iohexol in excretory urography. Results of drug monitoring [German]. *Fortschritte der Medizin* 1986;104:153–156.
7. Wolf GL, Arenson RL, Cross AP. A prospective trial of ionic vs. nonionic contrast agents in routine clinical practice: Comparison of adverse effects. *Invest Radiol* 1990;25:S20–S21.
8. Wolf GL. A prospective trial of ionic vs. nonionic contrast agents in rou-tine clinical practise: Comparison. Comparison of adverse effects. *AJR* 1989;152:939–944.
9. Hruby W, Stellamor K. Long-term results using a nonionic contrast medium: A report of clinical experiences [German]. *Rontgen-Blatter* 1987;40:73–77.
10. Brasch RC. Evidence supporting an antibody mediation of contrast media reactions. *Invest Radiol* 1980;15:529–532.
11. Lasser EC, Hang J, et al. Activation systems in contrast idiosyncrasy. *Invest Radiol* 1980;15:2–6.

12. Grainger RG. Intravascular contrast media—The past, the present and the future. *Br J Radiol* 1982;55:1–18.
13. Lalli AF. Contrast media reactions: Data analysis and hypothesis. *Radiology* 1980;134:1–12.
14. Ansell G, Tweedie MCK, Evans P, Couch L. The current status of reactions to intravenous contrast media. *Invest Radiol* 1980;1S:S32–S39.
15. Lalli AF. Contrast media deaths. *Australas Radiol* 1984;28:133–135.
16. Bochner BS, Lichtenstein LM. Anaphylaxis. *N Engl J Med* 1991;324 (25):1785–1790.
17. Byrd L, Sherman RL. Radiocontrast-induced acute renal failure: A clinical and pathophysiologic review. *Medicine* 1979;58:270–279.
18. Mudge GH. Nephrotoxicity of urographic radiocontrast drugs. *Kidney International* 1980;18:540–552.
19. Schwab SJ, Hlatky MA, Pieper KS, et al. Contrast nephrotoxicity: A randomized controlled trial of nonionic and an ionic radiographic contrast agent. *N Engl J Med* 1989;320:149–153.
20. Runge VM. *Clinical Magnetic Resonance Imaging.* JB Lippincott, Philadelphia; 1990, p. 504.
21. Goldstein HA, Kashanian FK, et al. Safety assessment of gadopentetate dimeglumine in U.S. clinical trials. *Radiology* 1990;174:17–23.

IMAGE-GUIDED PAIN MANAGEMENT
edited by P. S. Thomas.
Lippincott–Raven Publishers, Philadelphia © 1997

3

Sphenopalatine Ganglion

John J. Cambareri

Department of Anesthesiology, SUNY Health Science Center at Syracuse,
Syracuse, New York 13210

A great number of unusual signs and symptoms have been attributed to dysfunction of the sphenopalatine ganglion (synonyms: Meckel's g, pterygopalatine g, or sphenomaxillary g) and the nerves that pass through it. As summarized by Ruskin (12) the blockade of the ganglion has, over the last 100 years, been touted as a useful treatment for epilepsy, blindness, glaucoma, earache, migraine, asthma, angina, hiccup, low back pain, sciatica, menstrual pain, and hyperthyroidism. The block was so popular by the 1930s that Byrd and Byrd reported their experience with over 10,000 sphenopalatine ganglion blocks in 2,000 patients (4). In the following decades the block fell into disrepute and few controlled studies were done (18). More recently, blockade and ablation of the ganglion has been advocated for treatment of nicotine addiction (6), low back pain (1), generalized pain in the "difficult" patient (9), cluster headache and sphenopalatine neuralgia (3,5,10,13,15). Currently, sphenopalatine block or ablation for treatment of facial pain with signs associated with ipsilateral autonomic over-activity, i.e., cluster headache or sphenopalatine neuralgia, has enjoyed more widespread acceptance (14).

There is much confusion regarding the descriptions, pathogenesis, and treatment of unilateral facial pain, particularly when it is associated with ipsilateral autonomic over-activity (14). Terms and eponyms that illustrate this lack of consensus

27

include: sphenopalatine neuralgia, cluster headache, Sluder's syndrome, Horton's headache, histamine cephalgia, Charlin's syndrome, vidian headache, Vail's syndrome, and autonomic facial cephalgia. The two terms most commonly used are *sphenopalatine neuralgia* and *cluster headache* although controversy exists whether these represent different pathological processes or are, in fact, the same clinical entity (5).

The term sphenopalatine neuralgia was first coined by Sluder in 1909 (17) describing paroxysms of excruciating pain located behind one eye and associated with ipsilateral parasympathetic overactivity. Vasodilatation of the ipsilateral face with lacrimation and nasal congestion are characteristic features that may or may not precede the facial pain. Miosis and ptosis occur commonly.

Unlike migraine the pain begins with little or no warning and may awaken the patient from sleep. The pain quickly builds up in intensity and is described as sharp, knife-like, or throbbing. The attacks usually last from 30 minutes to 2 hours and may cease abruptly. Attacks occur in groups (clusters) that vary from 10 days to 3 months apart. Within each cluster paroxysms may occur 1 to 15 times per day.

The therapy (2,14) for acute attacks include the inhalation of 100% O_2 (60–70% effective after 10–15 min), intranasal dihydroergotamine (50% effective), or subcutaneous sumatriptan 6 mg (80% effective after 15 min).

There is no general consensus on the effectiveness of medical therapy for prevention of cluster headache (2,14). Medical prophylaxis may include chronic administration of lithium carbonate, methysergide, ergotamine tartrate (oral form currently unavailable in the US), calcium channel antagonists or high dose corticosteroids.

Blockage of the ganglion using local anesthetics during an attack is a useful tool to decide whether ablation of the ganglion would give pain relief. Unfortunately, surgical resection of the sphenopalatine ganglion, while helpful for many, is neither universally effective nor permanent (3,5,10,15). Radiofrequency (13) or alcohol ablation (2,7,14) of the ganglion is significantly less invasive and may be repeated as often as the pain recurs.

ANATOMY

The sphenopalatine ganglion is located in the pterygopalatine fossa; just posterior to the maxillary air sinus, lateral to the perpendicular plate of the palatine bone, and anterior to the medial plate of the pterygoid process. Posteriorly the foramen rotundum produces the maxillary nerve and the pterygoid (vidian) canal produces the nerve of the pterygoid canal. The ganglion is accessible laterally through the infratemporal fossa (percutaneously), inferiorly through the greater palatine foramen (intraoral), and medially through the sphenopalatine foramen (intranasal).

The sphenopalatine ganglion contains parasympathetic, sympathetic, and somatosensory nerves. Presynaptic parasympathetic fibers enter the ganglion from the facial nerve via the greater petrosal nerve and the nerve of the pterygoid canal. Secretomotor postsynaptic fibers are distributed to the nasal mucosa and the palatine and lacrimal glands. Somatosensory fibers from the maxillary nerve travel through the ganglion and innervate the palate and tonsil (greater and lesser palatine nn.) and the posterior two thirds of the nasal septum (nasopalatine n.). Sympathetic fibers from the carotid plexus travel to the ganglion via the deep petrosal nerve and the nerve of the pterygoid (vidian) canal and provide innervation to lacrimal glands and various blood vessels.

METHOD

Intranasal (Blind)

Sluder's (17) approach to sphenopalatine ganglion blockade was by using either a cocaine soaked cotton-tipped applicator or long needle directed through the naris along the lower border of the middle turbinate until the posterior wall of the nasopharynx was encountered. Depending on the concentration of local anesthetic and how close to the sphenopalatine foramen the applicator came the ganglion was usually anesthetized. This technique remains the most popular approach to the sphenopalatine ganglion despite it being an essentially blind block. This approach is not particularly useful for ablation of the ganglion due to difficulty placing the needle through the sphenopalatine foramen and into the ganglion reliably and the danger of sloughing of nasal mucosa.

Intraoral (Blind)

The ganglion can often be reached via the greater palatine foramen. In this technique the patient is placed supine with a pillow under their shoulders and neck extended. A small gauge needle is prepared by producing a 100° to 120° bend approximately 2 inches from the tip. The greater palatine foramen is palpated and the needle is inserted in a superior and slightly posterior direction for approximately 1.5 inches. A paresthesia to the palate is often obtained. Occasionally an infraorbital paresthesia is obtained indicating the tip of the needle has passed the ganglion and has touched the maxillary nerve. Once the needle is properly placed 0.2 ml (3) to 2 ml (8) of solution is injected. As in the intranasal approach, the successful placement of the needle in the ganglion may be difficult in inexperienced hands, and a poorly placed needle risks blockade of the maxillary nerve and slough of nasal mucosa.

Infratemporal (Image-Guided)

On a suitable radiolucent table, the patient is placed with the head in moderate extension. The midpoint of the zygoma is palpated and a small gauge needle (a 3.5 inch spinal needle works nicely) is inserted perpendicular to the skin until the

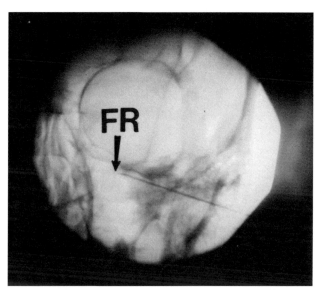

FIG. 1. Anterior-posterior (AP) view of the head showing correct placement of the needle in the sphenopalatine fossa. **FR** = foramen rotundum.

lateral plate of the pterygoid is encountered. The needle is withdrawn slightly and under fluoroscopy (anteroposterior view) redirected anteriorly and superiorly an additional 1 to 1.5 cm until the tip of the needle is seen immediately inferior to the foramen rotundum (Fig. 1). If bone is encountered, care should be taken so as not to force the needle through it into the maxillary or sphenoid sinus. The position of the needle is confirmed in the lateral view with the tip of the needle just anterior and inferior to the anterior wall of the sphenoid sinus (Fig. 2). Injection of 0.5 ml increments of solution, up to 2 ml total, will anesthetize the sphenopalatine ganglion and the nerves passing through it. The maxillary nerve may also be affected with the primary symptom being numbness in the infraorbital region. If a lytic block is desired, local anesthetic should be injected first and the patient evaluated as to extent of the block, including vision and skin over the face before any neurotoxic agents are administered.

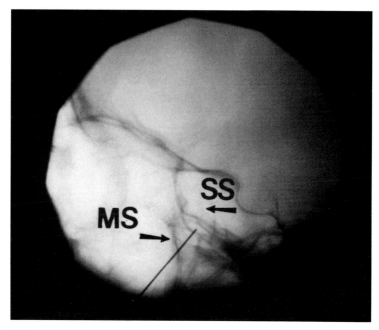

FIG. 2. Lateral view of the head showing needle tip just anterior and inferior to the sphenoid sinus. **SS** = anterior wall of the sphenoid sinus. **MS** = posterior wall of the maxillary sinus.

REFERENCES

1. Berger JJ, Pyles ST, Saga-Rumley SA. Does topical anesthesia of the sphenopalatine ganglion with cocaine or lidocaine relieve low back pain? *Anesth Analg* 1986;65:700–702.
2. Bonica JJ. *The management of pain, 2nd ed.* Lea and Febiger, Philadelphia; 1990:716–720, 810.
3. Brown LA. Mythical sphenopalatine ganglion neuralgia. *Southern Medical Journal* 1962;55:670–672.
4. Byrd H, Byrd W. Sphenopalatine phenomena: Present status of knowledge. *Arch Intern Med* 1930;46:1026–1038.
5. Cepero R, Miller RH, Bressler KL. Long-term results of sphenopalatine ganglioneurectomy for facial pain. *Am J Otolaryngol* 1987;8:171–174.
6. Henneberger JT, Menk EJ, Middaugh RE, Finstuen K. Sphenopalatine ganglion blocks for the treatment of nicotine addiction. *Southern Medical Journal* 1988;81:832–836.
7. Jurgens EH, Jurgens PE. Syndromes involving facial pain. In: *Facial pain, 2nd ed.* Alling CC and Mahan PE. Lea and Febiger, Philadelphia; 1977:227–236.

8. Katz J. *Atlas of regional anesthesia.* Appleton-Century-Croft; 1984:16–17.
9. Lebovits AH, Alfred H, Lefkowitz M. Sphenopalatine block: Clinical use in the pain management clinic. *Clin J Pain* 1990;6:131–136.
10. Meyer JS, Binns PM, Ericsson AD, Vulpe M. Sphenopalatine ganglionectomy for cluster headache. *Arch Otolaryng* 1970;92:475–484.
11. Prasanna A, Murthy PSN. Combined stellate ganglion and sphenopalatine ganglion block in acute herpes infection. *Clin J Pain* 1993;9:135–137.
12. Ruskin AP. Sphenopalatine (nasal) ganglion: Remote effects including "psychosomatic" symptoms, rage reaction, pain, and spasm. *Arch Phys Med Rehabil* 1979;60:353–359.
13. Salar G, Ori C, Iob I, Fiore D. Percutaneous thermocoagulation for sphenopalatine ganglion neuralgia. *Acta Neurochir (Wien)* 1987;84:24–28.
14. Schoenen J, de Noordhout AM. Headache. In: Wall PD, Melzack R, eds. *Textbook of pain, 3rd ed.* Churchill Livingstone, New York; 1994:495–521.
15. Sewall EC. Surgical removal of the sphenopalatine ganglion. *Ann Otol Rhino Laryngol* (Reprint of 1937 article.) 1992;101:285–292.
16. Silverman DG, Spencer RF, Kitahata LM, O'Connor TZ. Lack of effect of sphenopalatine ganglion block with intranasal lidocaine on submaximal effort tourniquet test pain. *Reg Anesth* 1993;19:356–360.
18. Waldman SD. Sphenopalatine ganglion block—80 years later. *Reg Anesth* 1993;18:274–276.
19. Sluder G. The anatomical and clinical relations of the sphenopalatine ganglion to the nose and its accessory sinuses. *New York J Med* 1909;8:293–298.

IMAGE-GUIDED PAIN MANAGEMENT
edited by P. S. Thomas.
Lippincott–Raven Publishers, Philadelphia © 1997

4

Glossopharyngeal Nerve Block

Paul H. Willoughby

Department of Anesthesiology, SUNY Health Science Center at Syracuse, Syracuse, New York 13210

CASE

A 65-year-old male presents with right-sided pharyngeal pain. One year ago, the patient was diagnosed with laryngeal cancer for which he refused surgery but accepted radiation therapy. The tumor has now regrown and the patient refuses surgery and radiation therapy. He is currently taking 200 mg of morphine a day. He describes his pain as a sharp, burning pain beginning in his right oropharynx and radiating to his ear. Our plan is a diagnostic glossopharyngeal nerve block for possible neurolytic block and/or neurosurgical decompression.

INTRODUCTION

The glossopharyngeal nerve emerges from the jugular foramen with the vagus nerve, the spinal accessory nerve, and the internal jugular vein. It travels posterior and medial to the styloid process just lateral to the internal carotid artery. The glossopharyngeal nerve provides sensation to the posterior third of the tongue, the oropharynx including the epiglottis, the fauces, and the pharynx to the esophagopharyngeal junction. It also provides chemoreceptors and baroreceptors at the carotid bulb.

Common indications for blockade include anesthesia for awake intubation, post tonsillectomy pain, and cancer pain.

These include carcinoma of the posterior third of the tongue and carcinoma of the pharynx. Other indications include glossopharyngeal neuralgia and to differentiate it from geniculate neuralgia (secondary to facial nerve and nervus intermedius). The former indications are easily achieved with an intraoral approach. However, for cancer pain where tumor and previous surgery may distort the anatomy, the extra oral route is preferred. As the vagus nerve, the spinal accessory nerve, the internal jugular vein and carotid artery lie in close proximity to the glossopharyngeal nerve, and the styloid process can be difficult to palpate or is abnormal in 5% of patients, it would seem advantageous to perform this block under radiological guidance (2,5,6).

TECHNIQUE FOR GLOSSOPHARYNGEAL BLOCK UNDER CT GUIDANCE

The patient is placed in the supine position and the head is tilted away from the side being blocked. A line is drawn from the angle of the mandible to the mastoid process. The spot for needle placement is marked at the midpoint of this line. Then the area is prepped with antiseptic and draped. The patient is placed inside the CT scanner and the laser localization light is placed across the spot marked previously. A scout film is taken and the anatomy is now defined (Fig. 1). The position of the glossopharyngeal nerve is seen. Its depth and position relative to the styloid process is noted. A 22-gauge blunt beveled needle is placed after subcutaneous infiltration with local anesthetic and guided in the same plane as the scout film (laser localization light) half the distance to the nerve. The CT is repeated to ensure accurate direction and then the needle is placed the appropriate distance (1 to 3 cm total distance from skin). The CT is taken again to document that the needle is close to and posterior to styloid process (Fig. 2). A small amount of radio opaque dye is injected to document the extent of the spread (Fig. 3). The local anesthetic or neurolytic agent is titrated in 0.1 cc increments until desired effect is achieved (typically 0.5-1.0 cc).

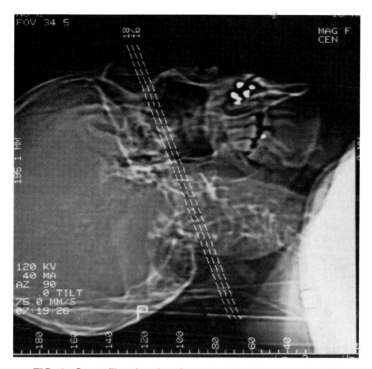

FIG. 1. Scout film showing the cuts to be taken on the CT.

DISCUSSION

Glossopharyngeal nerve block can have many complications. Due to the proximity of major vascular structures, intravascular injection, or necrosis of tissue may occur. The vagus and the spinal accessory nerve are usually also effected. Thus, the patient may lose the use of the ipsilateral trapezius muscle and be hoarse. The patient's blood pressure and heart rate may increase due to block of the baroreceptor afferent activity (4). The patient may also become more prone to hypoxemia due to block of chemoreceptor afferent fibers. Bilateral blockade would greatly increase the effects on heart rate, blood pressure, risks of hypoxemia as well as completely obliterate the gag reflex to touch in the pharynx (3).

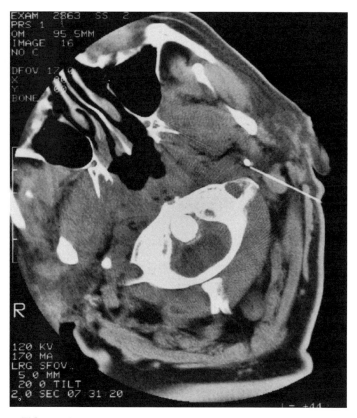

FIG. 2. Needle close to and posterior to the styloid process.

Utilizing computerized augmented tomography offers the distinct advantage of visualizing the location of the glossopharyngeal nerve itself and thus minimizing the amount of solution needed for effect. Hopefully this would minimize side effects and complications as well. The block can also be performed under x-ray guidance by defining the location of the styloid process and placing the needle relative to this landmark. Ultrasound has also been used to establish the location of the carotid artery and blocking the glossopharyngeal nerve as it passes superficially to this structure (1).

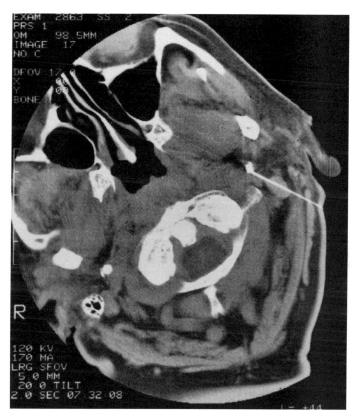

FIG. 3. Radio opaque dye in place.

REFERENCES

1. Bedder MD. Glossopharyngeal nerve block using ultrasound guidance: A case report of a new technique. *Regional Anesthesia* 1989;14:304–307.
2. Bonica JJ. Local anesthesia and regional blocks. In: Wall PD, Melzack R, eds. *Textbook of pain*. Churchill Livingstone, London; 1984.
3. Eisly JH, Jain SK. Circulatory and respiratory changes during unilateral and bilateral cranial nerve IX and X block in two asthmatics. *Clin Sci* 1971;40:117–125.
4. Fagius J, Wallin BG, Sundlof G, Nerhed C, Englesson S. Sympathetic outflow in man after anaesthesia of the glossopharyngeal and vagus nerves. *Brain* 1985;108:423–438.

5. Montgomery W, Cousins MJ. Aspects of the management of chronic pain illustrated by ninth nerve block. *Brit J Anaesth* 1972;44:383–385.
6. Murphy TM. Somatic blockade of head and neck. In: Cousins MJ, Bridenbough PO, eds. *Neural blockade in clinical anesthesia and management of pain.* JB Lippincott, Philadelphia, 1988.

IMAGE-GUIDED PAIN MANAGEMENT
edited by P. S. Thomas.
Lippincott–Raven Publishers, Philadelphia © 1997

5

Maxillary Nerve Block

Syed I. Hosain and P. Sebastian Thomas

*Department of Anesthesiology, SUNY Health Science Center at Syracuse,
Syracuse, New York 13210*

INDICATIONS

Anesthesiologists use a blockade of the maxillary nerve in the operating room for postoperative analgesia following surgery to the maxilla and face or for removal of teeth from the upper jaw. The block may be utilized diagnostically for isolated neuralgias and neuropathies of the maxillary nerve (3). These may arise from neoplasia, surgical injury, or trauma. The injection of alcohol may result in a post-injection neuritis. Our practice is to avoid this agent. However, phenol in a 2% or 4% solution can be used with much less risk of a post-injection neuritis (1). The phenol should be dissolved in glycerine to limit inadvertent spread.

ANATOMY

The second division of the trigeminal nerve contains sensory fibers and a few fibers which join the sphenopalatine ganglion (although functionally most of the fibers connected to the sphenopalatine ganglion arise from the facial nerve). Its branches can be divided as follows: intracranial, branches in the pterygopalatine fossa, infraorbital branches, and facial branches (4). The maxillary nerve gives sensory supply to dura of the middle cranial fossa, the skin of the face over the maxilla, around the inferior aspect of the eyes, and the lateral edge of the nose. The

41

terminal branch of the maxillary nerve forms the infraorbital nerve. The nerve arises from the middle of the trigeminal ganglion and exits the base of the skull through the foramen rotundum. It then crosses the pterygopalatine fossa and enters the orbit via the infraorbital fossa.

TECHNIQUE OF BLOCKADE

The patient is placed in the supine position with the head turned to the direction opposite to the side of the block. After aseptic preparation of the skin, the patient is asked to open his or her mouth and the coronoid notch is palpated. A finder needle is placed on the skin over the notch to locate the position of the coronoid notch. Then fluoroscopy in a lateral projection is used to confirm the position of the notch and to identify the midpoint of the zygoma. A 22-gauge 8-cm needle is inserted through the skin overlying the notch about 1 cm below the midpoint of the

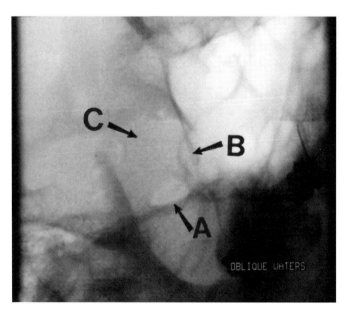

FIG. 1. Oblique waters view showing foramen ovale. **A**: Foramen ovale; **B**: Lateral pterygoid plate; **C**: Sphenoid bone.

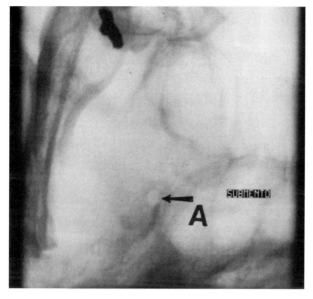

FIG. 2. Submento view showing foramen ovale; **A**: Foramen ovale.

arch of the zygoma in a slightly cephalic and medial direction so as to make contact with the lateral pterygoid plate (2) (Fig. 1, modified waters view). An oblique film taken from an antero-posterior position will help to confirm the position of the anterior edge of the lateral pterygoid plate. The needle is then repositioned so as to enter the pterygopalatine fossa. A fluoroscopic view taken in lateral projection will confirm the position of the needle (Fig. 2, submento view). The depth of the needle should be no more than 1 cm greater than the initial depth at which the lateral pterygoid plate was contacted.

After careful aspiration, 3 to 5 cc of local anesthetic may be injected. Figure 3 shows an axial cut of the CT scan demonstrating anatomy of the foramen ovale.

COMPLICATIONS OF BLOCK

The pterygopalatine fossa is a vascular region containing branches of the maxillary artery. Inadvertent intravascular injection is possible and also hematoma formation in the infra-

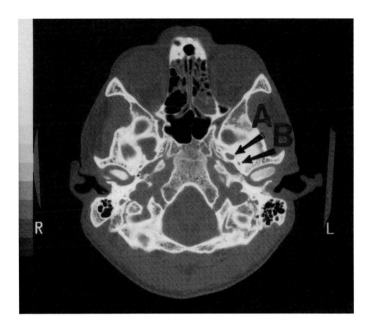

FIG. 3. Axial cut on the CT scan showing foramen ovale and foramen sphenosum; **A**: Foramen ovale; **B**: Foramen sphenosum.

orbital area. The patient should be warned of this possibility. Some spread of the local anesthetic into the orbit can occur resulting in partial anesthesia of the extra ocular muscles.

REFERENCES

1. Bonica JJ, Buckley FP, Moricca G, Murphy TM. Block of the ophthalmic, maxillary and mandibular nerves in neurolytic blockade and hypophysectomy. In: Bonica JJ, Loeser JD, Chapman CR, Fordyce WE, eds. *The management of pain, 2nd ed.* Lea and Febiger, Malvern and Beckenham, 1990.
2. Brown DL. Maxillary block. *Atlas of regional anesthesia.* WB Saunders Co., Philadelphia; 1992:141-146.
3. Murphy TM. somatic blockade of head and neck. In: Cousins MJ, Bridenbaugh PO, eds. *Neural blockade in clinical anesthesia and management of pain, 2nd ed.* JB Lippincott, Philadelphia; 1988:533–558.
4. Warwick R, Williams PL, eds. The maxillary nerve. *Gray's anatomy, 35th ed.* Longman Group, Edinburgh; 1978:1004–1007.

IMAGE-GUIDED PAIN MANAGEMENT
edited by P. S. Thomas.
Lippincott–Raven Publishers, Philadelphia © 1997

6

Mandibular Nerve Block

Syed I. Hosain and P. Sebastian Thomas

Department of Anesthesiology, SUNY Health Science Center at Syracuse, Syracuse, New York 13210

INDICATIONS

This block is utilized by anesthesiologists for selective analgesia of the mandible and teeth of the lower jaw. It is used by pain specialists in the diagnosis and treatment of isolated mandibular nerve neuralgias and neuropathies. These may arise from neoplasia, surgical injury, or trauma. The nerve is accessible for both techniques involving local anesthetics and cryotherapy. The injection of alcohol may result in a post-injection neuritis. Our practice is to avoid this agent. However, phenol in a 2% or 4% solution can be used with much less risk of a post-injection neuritis. The phenol should be dissolved in glycerine to limit inadvertent spread (1).

ANATOMY

The mandibular nerve supplies innervation to the teeth and gums of the lower jaw, part of the auricle, the lower lip, lower part of the face, and the muscles of mastication. The mandibular nerve is the largest division of the trigeminal nerve. It is composed of a sensory root and a motor root. The nerve then enters the infratemporal fossa (3,4). The lateral wall of the infratemporal fossa is the ramus of the mandible and coronoid process of the mandible, in the anterior portion

45

of the fossa the lateral pterygoid plate forms the medial wall and posteriorly the fossa is bounded by the constrictor muscles of the pharynx. A needle introduced through the coronoid process across the infratemporal fossa can be used to block the third division nerve.

TECHNIQUE OF THE BLOCK

The patient is placed in the supine position with the head turned to the opposite side of the block. The side of the face is prepared and the patient is asked to open his/her mouth slightly. The midpoint of the zygomatic arch is found. A skin wheal is raised with local anesthetic just below this point (2). The location of the coronoid notch should be confirmed fluoroscopically with a lateral view of the skull. A 3-inch needle is inserted in a medial direction through the coronoid notch across the

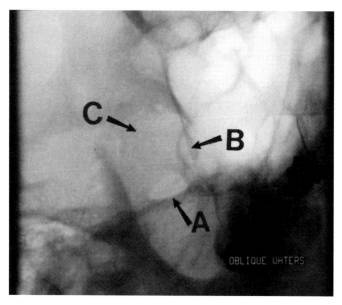

FIG. 1. Oblique waters view showing foramen ovale. **A**: Foramen ovale; **B**: Lateral pterygoid plate; **C**: Sphenoid bone.

infratemporal fossa toward the lateral pterygoid plate. The depth of the lateral pterygoid plate is usually about 2 inches. An AP view of the skull can help in confirming the depth of the lateral pterygoid plate (Fig. 1). The needle is then directed posteriorly in small steps so as to walk off the posterior aspect of the lateral pterygoid plate toward the auditory meatus. Figure 2 shows submento view of the foramen ovale. A paraesthesia should be obtained in the third division distribution. The depth of the needle should be no more than 2 1/4 inches. Placing the needle deeper than this will risk puncturing the superior constrictor muscle of the pharynx. A small volume of local anesthetic up to 3 cc is required to produce anesthesia of this nerve. Our own practice is to use 0.25% bupivacaine 1 cc to 3 cc. Phenol may be used in a volume of up to 1 cc after the injection of a radio contrast dye. As in the chapter on Axillary Nerve block, Figure 3 shows an axial cut of the CT scan demonstrating anatomy of the foramen ovale.

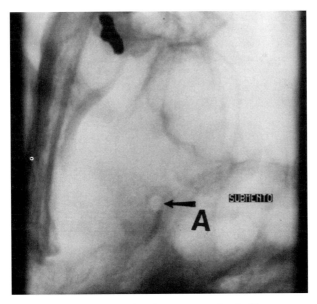

FIG. 2. Submento view showing foramen ovale; **A**: Foramen ovale.

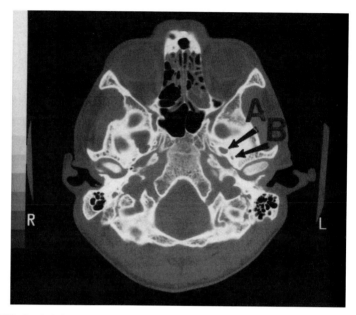

FIG. 3. Axial cut on the CT scan showing foramen ovale and foramen sphenosum; **A**: Foramen ovale; **B**: Foramen sphenosum.

COMPLICATIONS

These include inadvertent injection of local anesthetic into the cerebrospinal fluid through the foramen ovale; very small doses of local anesthetic can produce unconsciousness. The path of the needle is through a highly vascular region and there is a risk of hematoma formation. If the needle is inserted through the superior constrictor of the pharynx, it may risk introducing bacteria into an area of the meninges.

REFERENCES

1. Bonica JJ, Buckley FP, Moricca G, Murphy TM. Block of the ophthalmic, maxillary and mandibular nerves in neurolytic blockade and hypophysectomy. In: Bonica JJ, Loeser JD, Chapman CR, Fordyce WE eds. *The management of pain, 2nd ed.* Lea and Febiger, Malvern and Beckenham, 1990.

2. Brown DL. Mandibular nerve. In: *Atlas of regional anesthesia.* WB Saunders, Philadelphia; 1992:147–152.
3. Murphy TM. Somatic blockade of head and neck. In: Cousins MJ, Bridenbaugh PO, eds. *Neural blockade in clinical anesthesia and management of pain, 2nd ed.* JB Lippincott, Philadelphia; 1988:533–558.
4. Warwick R, Williams PL, eds. The mandibular nerve. *Gray's anatomy, 35th ed.* Longman Group, Edinburgh; 1978:1007–1010.

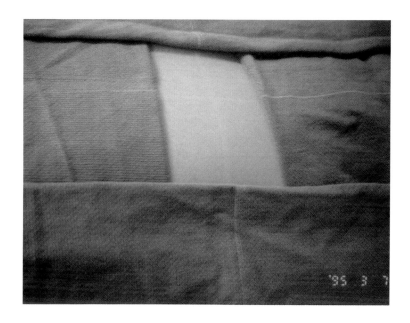

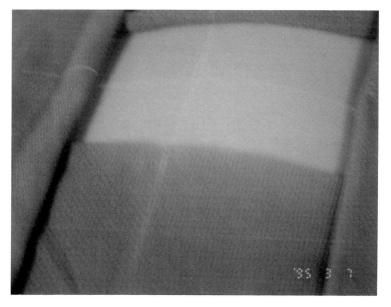

Color Plate. Laser markers projected from the CT scanner to denote the midline and axial level.

IMAGE-GUIDED PAIN MANAGEMENT
edited by P. S. Thomas.
Lippincott–Raven Publishers, Philadelphia © 1997

7

Trigeminal Nerve Block

Pramod Yadhati, Syed I. Hosain, and P. Sebastian
Thomas

*Department of Anesthesiology, SUNY Health Science Center at Syracuse,
Syracuse, New York 13210*

INDICATIONS

These can be divided into diagnostic and therapeutic indications. There are three important therapeutic indications:

1. Herpetic neuralgia in the trigeminal division
2. Tic douloureux
3. Neoplasms involving the trigeminal ganglion.

ANATOMY OF THE TRIGEMINAL GANGLION

The gasserian or trigeminal ganglion is located in a recess of bone known as *Meckel's cave* (3). Meckel's cave lies in the apex of the petrous temporal bone. It contains a fold of the dura in which there is cerebrospinal fluid in direct continuity with the rest of the CSF. The gasserian ganglion is reached through the foramen ovale through which exits the mandibular branch of the trigeminal nerve (Figs. 1 and 2). Anteriorly and superiorly is the foramen rotundum through which the maxillary division of the trigeminal nerve exits. The medial relations of the ganglion are the internal carotid artery and the posterior cavernous sinus; the latter containing the third, fourth, fifth, and sixth cranial nerve. The superior relation is the temporal lobe and laterally the arch of the zygoma. Any structures in close

51

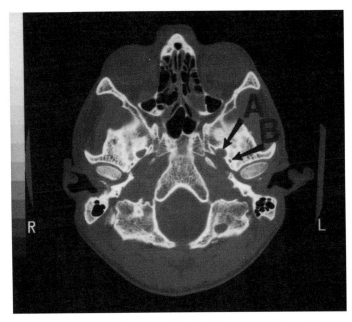

FIG. 1. Axial cut of the CT scan showing foramen ovale and foramen sphenosum. **A**: foramen ovale; **B**: foramen sphenosum.

relationship to the ganglion may be damaged or may be sites for inadvertent injection. Spread of injectate in the cerebrospinal fluid (CSF) could in principle result in remote central nervous system effects.

TECHNIQUE OF PERFORMING THE BLOCK

The face is an area of the body with special importance for most people thus any procedure around the face is accompanied by considerable apprehension. This is no less true for the blockade of the trigeminal ganglion. A small dose of narcotic may be employed to sedate the patient prior to the performance of the block. The patient should be appropriately monitored with pulse oximetry and also blood pressure measurements.

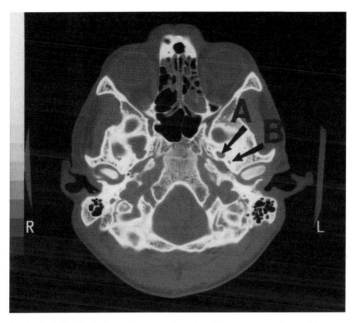

FIG. 2. Axial cut of the CT scan showing foramen ovale and foramen sphenosum. **A**: foramen ovale; **B**: foramen sphenosum.

The patient is placed supine on the fluoroscopy table. A plane image in the modified Water's view and a second image in the submental view are obtained. In these images, it should be possible to identify the major landmarks of the base of the skull. The entry point of the needle will be approximately 1 to 1.5 cm posterior and lateral to the lateral margin of the mouth (1,2). The point of entry will be in the cheek above the second molar, however, the needle should not pass through the mouth. Then a 22-gauge 8-cm needle is directed in line with the pupil with the patient gazing forward and toward the mid point of the zygomatica arch. A lateral image of the skull will help to judge this angle correctly. Figures 3 and 4 show the modified waters view and the submento view to accurately locate the foramen ovale. The position of the needle may initially impinge on the roof of the infratemporal fossa. Often,

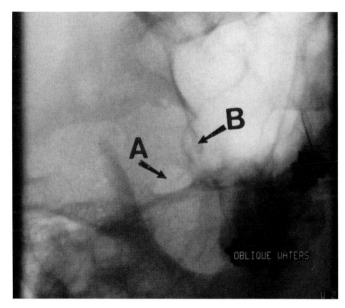

FIG. 3. Oblique waters view showing foramen ovale. **A**: Foramen ovale; **B**: Lateral pterygoid plate.

the needle will have to be redirected in a more lateral, less cephalad direction.

A paraesthesia in the maxillary division may be obtained if the needle is placed in close proximity to the ganglion. Frequently, however, a paraesthesia in the mandibular division occurs which may be elicited in the infratemporal fossa before the needle slips into Meckel's cave.

The needle should not be advanced more than 1 cm into Meckel's cave. After careful negative aspiration tests for CSF and blood, the local anesthetic or neurolytic agent is injected. This injection is made in 0.25 cc aliquots; bupivacaine 0.25% is a suitable drug. A total volume of 0.75 cc to 1.0 cc is sufficient. Alcohol and phenol have been used as neurolytic agents in this block. Neurolysis should always be preceded by a local anesthetic injection to confirm the effects of the block.

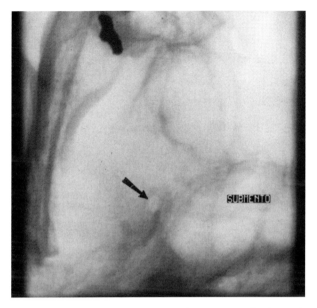

FIG. 4. Submental view showing foramen ovale *(arrow).*

COMPLICATIONS

The close proximity of the internal carotid artery, cranial nerves, and the CSF bathing the gasserian ganglion make this an extremely hazardous procedure in which meticulous attention to detail is vital. Tiny amounts of local anesthetic can render the patient unconscious and requiring cardiorespiratory support. The spread of neurolytic solutions can damage adjacent cranial nerves and render the patient temporarily unconscious. Hyperbaric solutions may spill over onto the 6th, 8th, 9th, 10th, 11th, and 12th cranial nerves.

Special mention is made here of complications related to the injection of neurolytic agents. The most important complication related to the injection of alcohol or phenol is of course anesthesia dolorosa. The injection of these agents should be reserved for patients not able to undergo neurosurgical procedures such as microvascular decompression or balloon gangliolysis. Other important complications include trigeminal motor weakness, corneal ulceration, and keratitis. Spread of the neurolytic agent in the cerebrospinal fluid is a potentially devastating complication.

REFERENCES

1. Bonica JJ, Buckley FP, Moricca G, Murphy TM. Gasserian ganglion block in neurolytic blockade and hypophysectomy. In: Bonica JJ, Loeser JD, Chapman CR, Fordyce WE, eds. *The management of pain, 2nd ed.* Lea and Febiger, Malvern and Beckenham, 1990.
2. Murphy TM. Somatic blockade of head and neck. In: Cousins MJ, Bridenbaugh PO, eds. *Neural blockade in clinical anesthesia and management of pain, 2nd ed.* JB Lippincott, Philadelphia; 1988:533–558.
3. Warwick R, Williams PL, eds. The trigeminal nerve in neurology. *Gray's anatomy, 35th ed.* Longman Group, Edinburgh; 1978.

IMAGE-GUIDED PAIN MANAGEMENT
edited by P. S. Thomas.
Lippincott–Raven Publishers, Philadelphia © 1997

8

Percutaneous Balloon Compression of the Trigeminal Ganglion-Technique

James W. Holsapple

Department of Neurological Surgery, SUNY Health Science Center at Syracuse, Syracuse, New York 13210

Percutaneous balloon compression (PBC) of the trigeminal ganglion is an effective and safe method of treating trigeminal neuralgia. The procedure in its present form is a percutaneous adaptation of the method described by Taarnjoh in the 1950s (4,5). Series data indicate that PBC carries little risk and is highly effective (2). The procedure is also an attractive option for patients for whom open microvascular decompression carries significant risk, such as in the elderly.

PATIENT SELECTION

PBC of the trigeminal ganglion is an effective therapy for patients with medically intractable trigeminal neuralgia. Patients with facial pain well managed with medication should not undergo a procedure of this type. As is often the case, however, many elderly patients experience recurrent severe bouts of facial pain requiring the use of either high doses of medication (Tegretol) and/or analgesics. The patients who are experiencing significant side effects from medications or overall ineffective management of their pain over a period of many weeks or months should be considered for operative therapy. It

57

remains controversial whether or not such patients are best treated by open decompression of the trigeminal nerve, percutaneous compression of the trigeminal nerve, or other ablative techniques. There is, of course, no single best choice and therapy needs to be customized.

PBC of the trigeminal ganglion appears to be safe and effective in patients of all ages, but is particularly useful in the elderly who may not wish to undergo craniotomy. The procedure requires exposure to a brief period of general anesthesia and a very low operative morbidity. Prior to balloon compression of the trigeminal ganglion, patients undergo MRI and CT scanning of the brain and skull base to rule out the presence of a compressive lesion of the trigeminal nerve. In such instances, PBC of trigeminal ganglion may or may not be safe or indicated. Such lesions are, however, rare.

OPERATIVE TECHNIQUE

The technique of PBC of the trigeminal ganglion has been well described previously and the reader is referred to the report by Mullin and Lictor (2) and Mullin (3). Provided here is a description of the procedure as it is performed at our institution and reflects only minor alterations in the procedure described by Mullin (3). The objective of the procedure is to place a balloon catheter through the foramen ovale into the vicinity of the trigeminal ganglion and compress the ganglion.

The patient is taken to a fluoroscopic suite, IVs placed, and general anesthesia induced. The chart is meticulously rechecked for the laterality of the pain. The patient is intubated and the endotracheal tube is placed against the opposing corner of the mouth. The arms are secured at the patient's side and the neck placed in extension with the occiput laid to rest on foam pads. A fluoroscopic submental vertex view of the skull is obtained. The head is rotated 10° to 30° away from the side of pain and the foramen ovale visualized. The foramen appears as an oval feature of the skull base just above the upper edge of the mandible with its long axis oriented roughly medial laterally. A point roughly 1 cm lateral and above the corner of the mouth on the affected side is then marked with a Kelly clamp over the foramen ovale. It is usually the case that this point and the foramen ovale are joined by a line roughly perpendicular to the floor. The face is then prepped with Septisol and a small field created with sterile towels. The fluoroscope source is draped with sterile cover. Items are prepared as follows: A #4 Fogarty catheter is then filled with Metrizamide and the balloon gently inflated to 0.8 cc. Care is taken to gently remove air from the balloon and the catheter. The catheter is then affixed to a 1 cc syringe which can be screw fastened. Again, the balloon is test inflated. If air is present in the balloon, it is gently tapped out and removed and the syringe reattached. With the balloon deflated, the Fogarty catheter is placed into a 14-gauge spinal needle and adjusted so that the proximal cuff to the balloon lies just beyond the bevel of the needle. The proximal portion of the catheter is then marked with a folded Steri-strip at the needle hub to indicate this depth. Care must be taken to be sure that the entire balloon lies just beyond the bevel of the needle. If this is not the case, the inflated balloon may rupture *in situ*. The Fogarty catheter is then removed from the trocar and the stylette replaced.

A 10-cc syringe is then filled with normal saline and attached to an 18-gauge needle. Under fluoroscopic control in the submental vertex view, the needle is directed through the previously chosen interpoint on the face and directed toward the foramen ovale. The needle, under optimal conditions, should be passed roughly perpendicular to the floor to the examination room to its full depth (roughly 2.5 cm) (Fig. 1B). It is slowly withdrawn and the track infiltrated with saline.

The 14-gauge spinal needle is then directed through the same puncture site toward the foramen ovale under constant fluoroscopy. The primary operator should be wearing radiopague gloves and is otherwise fully gowned and shielded for x-ray exposure. The needle is directed through the subbuccal tissue toward the foramen ovale in several steps. Eventually the needle engages dense tissue at the entrance of the foramen ovale. Before engaging the needle further and through the foramen ovale, it is important that the tip enter the foramen as close as

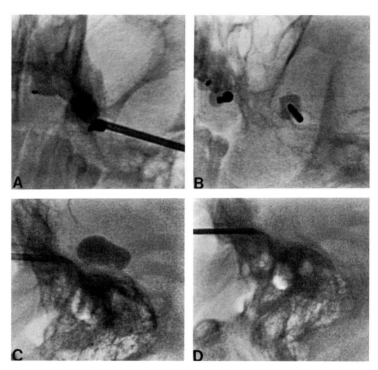

FIG. 1. **A**: Submental vertex view, partial injection, Fogarty catheter balloon. **B**: Submental vertex view, spinal needle engaged in foramen ovale. **C**: Lateral view, full volume injection balloon catheter. **D**: Lateral view, spinal needle engaged within the foramen ovale. Needle tip along floor of middle fossa. Balloon catheter not visible. Balloon uninflated.

possible to its mid-point. Once this has been confirmed, the needle is gently advanced several millimeters against moderate resistance. Although expected, there is usually no "pop" which indicates that the spinal needle has made its way beyond the foramen ovale into the middle cranial fossa. The needle is released and the fluoroscope rotated 90° to obtain a lateral view of the skull base (see Fig. 1D). When optimally placed, the trocar needle tip should be located just along the inner floor of the skull base and middle fossa. It is very important not to drive the needle deeper than this point, but it is equally important that the needle be engaged within the hatchway of the foramen ovale.

The inner stylette of the needle is removed and the balloon catheter placed inside to the previously marked depth. In some instances, the Fogarty catheter can be faintly seen on the fluoro-scopic lateral image, but its appearance should not be counted on to ascertain catheter placement. The catheter is then injected and the balloon inflated to a volume of 0.4 cc (see Fig. 1A). As this is done, the balloon can be seen on the fluoroscope as it fills with Metrizamide. The initial injection is done slowly at 0.1 mL incre-ments (3) and the configuration of the balloon observed. If the balloon does not lie beyond the foramen ovale, a "napkin ring waist" will appear. The balloon should be deflated and the catheter advanced 1 to 2 mm and the balloon reinflated. If, how-ever, the balloon assumes the configuration of a "pear" with its narrow end distal, the balloon is likely to be in good position (see Fig. 1C). It has been our practice to inflate the balloon to a vol-ume of 0.4 cc for a period of roughly 45 s. For an additional 15 to 45 s the balloon is gradually inflated to higher volumes in 0.1 mL steps until either a total volume of 0.7 cc or excessive resis-tance to further injection is sensed by the primary operator. We have preferred to stage the compression in this "low volume/high volume" stepwise fashion to assure that in the event of balloon rupture at higher volumes, the patients have received a substan-tial dose of low volume compression of the trigeminal ganglion.

Following 45 to 90 s of compression, the balloon is deflated and the Fogarty catheter and trocar removed together. A sponge is placed over the puncture site and pressure held for 10 to 15 minutes. There is usually very little bleeding from the puncture site and following direct compression, can be dressed with a Band-Aid. Patients are taken out of extension and allowed to recover from general anesthesia.

POSTOPERATIVE CARE

Because most patients treated in this manner are elderly, we have opted to keep them in the hospital overnight for observa-tion. If the procedure has been effective, the patients usually report dense analgesia over the 2nd and 3rd division of the trigeminal nerve on the operative side and usually the absence of their typical face pain if it was present just prior to the procedure. The morning following surgery, the patients are re-examined. If the face remains unswollen and there are no neurologic findings, the patients are discharged for home. They are instructed to continue taking Tegretol at 1/2 the prior dose.

RESULTS

The efficacy of this procedure has been well described (2,3). In his follow-up evaluation of 100 patients, Mullin reported (2) no major complications. Eighty percent of patients who completed 5-year follow-up have experienced no recurrence of face pain (3). Similar results have been reported elsewhere (1).

SUMMARY

PCB of the trigeminal ganglion is a relatively simple and effective method of treating trigeminal neuralgia which is proven refractory to other methods of treatment. The majority of patients remain free of their facial pain 5 years after the procedure. The procedure is pain free and it is a relatively safe alternative to direct open microvascular decompression of the trigeminal nerve. The procedure, therefore, represents a desirable option in the elderly patients or patients who face significant medical risk for sustained general anesthesia and craniotomy. The procedure does require, however, the coordination of an experienced anesthesia, radiographic, and neurosurgical team. It cannot be stressed enough that the familiarity of the primary operator and radiographic technician with the appearance of the skull base and foramen ovale is essential.

REFERENCES

1. Belbar CF, Rak RA. Balloon compression rhizolysis in the surgical management of trigeminal neuralgia. *Neurosurg* 1987;20(6):908–913.
2. Mullin S, Lichtor T. Percutaneous microcompression of the trigeminal ganglion for trigeminal neuralgia. *J Neurosurg* 1983;59:1007–1012.
3. Mullin S. Percutaneous microcompression of the trigeminal ganglion. In: Rovit R, Murali R, Janetta PJ, eds. *Trigeminal neuralgia*:137–144.

4. Sheldon CH, Pudenz RH, Freshwater B, Crue BL. Compression rather than decompression for trigeminal neuralgia. *J Neurosurg* 1955;12:123–126.
5. Taarnjoh P. Decompression of the trigeminal root and the posterior part of the ganglion as treatment for trigeminal neuralgia. Preliminary communication. *J Neurosurg* 1952;9:288–290.

IMAGE-GUIDED PAIN MANAGEMENT
edited by P. S. Thomas.
Lippincott–Raven Publishers, Philadelphia © 1997

9

X-Ray-Guided Cervical Epidural Block

David G. Fellows

*Department of Anesthesiology, SUNY Health Science Center at Syracuse,
Syracuse, New York 13210*

INDICATIONS

The major indication for cervical epidural steroid block is for the treatment of pain secondary to nerve root irritation. The use of epidural steroids to treat nerve root irritation secondary to herniated intervertebral discs is well documented (4,6). Epidural steroid blocks for diagnoses other than herniated disks is debatable (1,2). It is my opinion that cervical epidural steroids can be of assistance in cases of spinal stenosis and degenerative disc disease even if they only achieve temporary pain relief that allows the patient to enter in a program to improve their biomechanics and thus reduce their overall pain. Certainly, well-controlled prospective studies in this area are needed.

ANATOMY

The anatomy of the epidural space is well-described in several excellent regional anesthesia/pain texts (3,5). Here, the epidural space in the cervical region is very thin. The posterior–anterior width of the cervical epidural space is 1.5 to 2.0 mm (2). The thinness of the cervical epidural space requires meticulous attention to technique while performing a cervical epidural block.

EQUIPMENT

At SUNY Health Science Center at Syracuse, the preferred needle for cervical epidural blockade is an 18-gauge blunt tip needle, shown in Figure 1. The blunt tip needle has the advantage of making dural puncture less likely as no cutting surface can contact the dura. Additionally, in the advent of dural puncture or nerve root contact, the blunt tip is less likely to injure neural tissue. Because the needle is so blunt, an introducer is required to advance the needle beyond the skin and subcutaneous tissues.

PROCEDURE

After IV placement, the patient is positioned prone on the fluoroscopic table. The patient's arms are allowed to dangle off the table perpendicular to the floor. This allows a lateral x-ray

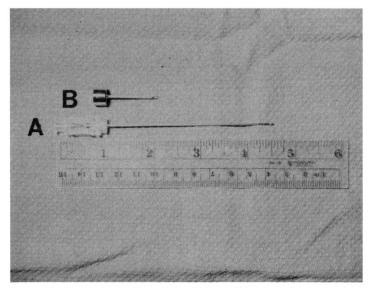

FIG. 1. 18-gauge blunt tip needle **(A)**, and introducer **(B)**.

to be taken if needed. The patient is instructed to flex his neck in a chin-to-chest manner.

Often, a soft roll under the chest is required for the patient to assume this position comfortably. The vertebra prominens (C7) is palpated and the desired level of entry is then determined. This level is confirmed by fluoroscopy.

Following local anesthesia to the skin, the introducer needle is advanced and seated in the ligament flavum using a midline approach. Midline position of the introducer is confirmed by fluoroscopy (Fig. 2). Proper midline placement is essential to avoid nerve root paresthesia. A syringe is attached to the blunt tip epidural needle and advanced 1 mm at a time until the epidural space is identified by the loss of resistance technique. Gentle aspiration is applied to the needle to ensure lack of cerebrospinal fluid (CSF). If doubt exists as to needle placement, fluoroscopy is used to determine position. If difficulty arises, an AP view is obtained to ensure the needle tip remains midline. A lateral view is then obtained to evaluate needle depth (Fig. 3). The epidural space is correctly located when the nee-

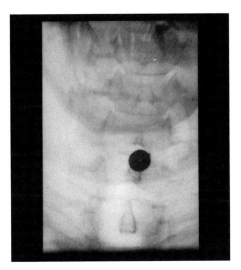

FIG. 2. PA view of the cervical spine showing introducer needle in midline position.

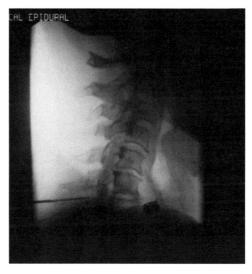

FIG. 3. Lateral view showing needle in the epidural space.

dle tip is seen to be just at the anterior rim of the spinous process. If a false loss of resistance is suspected, a lateral view showing shallow needle placement will confirm the suspicion. In difficult cases, the needle position can be continuously checked on lateral films to ensure that the loss of resistance felt represents needle placement in the epidural space. Upon correct placement, 80 mg of depomedrol mixed in 1 to 4 mL of 0.25% bupivacaine is injected through the needle. At SUNY Health Science Center, a series of up to three blocks spaced 2 weeks apart will be performed.

CASE REPORT

The patient was a 45-year-old female who, 2 weeks prior to referral to the pain clinic, awoke from sleep with severe pain in her neck and right arm. The patient reported that the pain was throbbing, aching, and shooting. The patient also complained of numbness in her right fourth and fifth fingers. There was no history of trauma. The patient had seen her primary care physician and an MRI of her neck was obtained. This revealed a C6–C7 disc herniation to the right side. The patient was started on physical therapy which she could not complete as it severely increased her pain. The patient had no complaints of bowel, bladder, or lower extremity problems.

The patient had no allergies, and review of systems, past medical and surgical histories were negative. Her only medication was Tylenol #4. On physical exam, the patient was essentially healthy. Her neck motion was limited in all directions secondary to pain. Cranial nerves were grossly intact. There were no abnormalities in gait, speech, or in her lower extremities.

The patient's neck was diffusely tender to palpation. Deep tendon reflexes were intact and equal bilaterally. There was a hyperesthesia noted in the right C7–C8 dermatomes on the right. Sensory to pinprick was intact. There were no temperature, color, or sudomotor changes noted.

The patient underwent two cervical epidural blocks as described previously. She received 2 mL of 0.25% marcaine and 80 mg of depomedrol with each block. Two weeks following her second block, the patient reported 80% relief of her pain. At this point, the patient elected to return to physical therapy and was discharged from the pain clinic's care.

REFERENCES

1. Benzon H. Epidural steroids. In: PP Raj, ed. *Practical management of pain, 2nd ed.* Mosby Year Book, St. Louis; 1992:820.
2. Cheng PA. Anatomical and clinical aspects of epidural anesthesia. *Current Res Anes Analg* 1963;42:392.
3. Cousins MJ, Bridenbaugh PO, eds. *Neural blockage in clinical anesthesia and management of pain, 2nd ed.* JB Lippincott, Philadelphia; 1988.
4. Dilke, TFW, Burry HC, Grahame R. Extradural corticosteroid injection in management of lumbar nerve root compression. *Brit Med J* 1973;2: 635–637.
5. Raj PP, ed. *Practical management of pain, 2nd ed.* Mosby Year Book, St. Louis; 1992.
6. White AH, Derby R, Wynne G. Epidural injections for the diagnosis and treatment of low back pain. *Spine* 1980;5:78–86.

IMAGE-GUIDED PAIN MANAGEMENT
edited by P. S. Thomas.
Lippincott–Raven Publishers, Philadelphia © 1997

10

Continuous Axillary Brachial Plexus Block

Paul H. Willoughby

Department of Anesthesiology, SUNY Health Science Center at Syracuse, Syracuse, New York 13210

CASE HISTORY

The patient is a 40-year-old female with a history of reflex sympathetic dystrophy of the right hand who has suffered a fracture of the right wrist. She is scheduled for open reduction and internal fixation of the right wrist. Anesthetic plan: axillary block with catheter placement and x-ray confirmation for postoperative pain management.

INTRODUCTION

Placement of an axillary catheter for continuous and intermittent brachial plexus blockade was initially described by Selander in 1977 (9). Indications for placement include intraoperative anesthesia in cases that may have a long duration, post-operative pain relief, prolonged sympathetic block in patients with vasoconstrictive disease for wound healing (7), arterial vasospasm, traumatic amputation, and pain relief during physical therapy in an extremely painful extremity. The aforementioned patient is also at risk for exacerbation of her underlying reflex sympathetic dystrophy. Complications of this procedure include infection (3), intravascular injection, possible nerve damage from paresthesia (10), venous insufficiency

(8), vascular insufficiency (5), and proximal blockade (Horner's syndrome; 4). Contraindications for blockade include patient refusal, local infection, and bleeding diathesis. Contraindications of contrast medium placement for confirmation of catheter placement include known allergy to contrast medium and iodine allergy.

METHOD

Using the classic Selander positioning and insertion technique, the patient is positioned supine and the arm is abducted to almost 90° and the elbow is flexed and rotated superiorly. The axilla is shaved (if necessary), prepped with antiseptic, and draped. The axillary artery is palpated below the insertion of the pectoralis major and subcutaneous local anesthesia is administered (1 to 2 cc) at this site. A small incision is made through the dermis but superficial to the artery with an 18-gauge needle. An 18-gauge catheter on a 20-gauge bullet tip needle is inserted at a 30° angle to the skin in the direction of the axilla toward the artery. When the neurovascular sheath is penetrated, a snap can often be felt. If a snap is not felt, either a paresthesia should be sought or a neurostimulator can be used. The needle is advanced toward the axilla slightly to ensure that the catheter is in the sheath. Then the catheter is advanced and the needle is removed. X-ray or fluoroscopic confirmation can then be obtained by injecting 2 cc of contrast medium via the placed catheter and visualizing the tubular space (Figs. 1 and 2). If the musculocutaneous nerve needs to be assuredly blocked, a longer catheter can be inserted through the 18-gauge catheter and confirmed with x-ray as just described.

Recently, a perivenous technique has been suggested by Pham-Dang (6). In this modification of the Selander technique, the patient is positioned as before but instead of identifying the axillary artery by palpation, the axillary vein is identified fluoroscopically by infusing small increments of intravenous contrast distally. Once identified, the needle is aimed at the axillary vein and the catheter is threaded under fluoroscopic guidance.

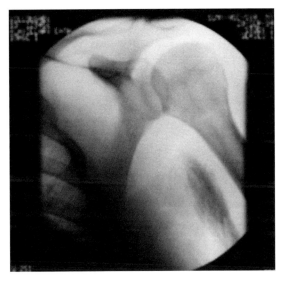

FIG. 1. PA view showing the spread of the dye in the axillary sheath.

This technique would offer advantages in patients with difficult anatomy (obese patients, etc.). However, an intravenous catheter must be placed distally and this may be difficult in patients with sympathetically mediated pain or trauma in this region.

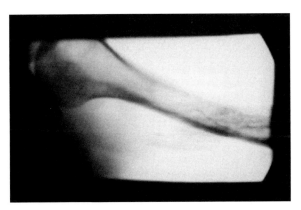

FIG. 2. Lateral view showing the spead of the dye in the axillary sheath.

Another method of achieving brachial plexus block via a catheter but without entering the neurovascular sheath has been suggested by Ang (1). With this method the patient is positioned and prepped as before and the site of insertion is 40 mm below the axilla, medial to the biceps muscle where the author states that the median nerve is easily palpable. The needle is then directed parallel to the median nerve, 20° from the skin in the direction of the axilla. The catheter is then placed in the space adjacent to the neurovascular bundle outside the sheath. Whereas the author reports a high success rate (98%), onset time of nerve blockade is increased.

DISCUSSION

Given the low success rate of placing an axillary catheter by the feel of the snap (as low as 56%), methods that increase the success rate of placement have been sought. Although eliciting a paresthesia or using a neurostimulator can increase the success rate, they are not 100%. By using radiological guidance, there is a better chance that the catheter will be placed correctly the first time.

REFERENCES

1. Ang ET, Lassale B, Goldfarb G. Continuous axillary brachial plexus block—A clinical and anatomical study. *Anesth Analg* 1984;63:680–684.
2. Baranowski AP, Pither CE. A comparison of three methods of brachial plexus anaesthesia. *Anaesthesia* 1990;45:362–365.
3. Greene ER. Intravascular injection of local anesthetic after venipuncture of axillary vein during attempted brachial plexus block. *Anesth Analg* 1986;65:421.
4. Lennon RL, Gammel S. Horner's Syndrome associated with brachial plexus anesthesia using an axillary catheter. *Anesth Analg* 1992;74:311–319.
5. Merrill DG, Brodsky JB, Hentz RV. Vascular insufficiency following axillary block of the brachial plexus. *Anesth Analg* 1981;60:162–164.
6. Pham-Dang C, Meunier JF, Poirier P, Kick O, Bourreli B, Touchais S, Le Corre P, Pinaud M. A new axillary approach for continuous brachial plexus block. A clinical and anatomic approach. *Anesth Analg* 1995;81:686–693.

7. Randalls B. Continuous brachial plexus blockade, a technique that uses an axillary catheter to allow successful skin grafting. *Anaesthesia* 1990; 45:143–144.
8. Restelli L, Pinciroli D, Conoscente F, Cammelli F. Insufficient venous drainage following axillary approach to brachial plexus blockade. *Brit J Anaesth* 1984;56:1051–1053.
9. Selander D. Catheter technique in axillary plexus block, presentation of a new method. *Acta Anaesthes Scandinavia* 1977;21:324–329.
10. Selander D, Edshage S, Wolf T. Paresthesia or no paresthesia? Nerve lesions after axillary blocks. *Acta Anaesthes Scandinavia* 1979;23: 27–33.

IMAGE-GUIDED PAIN MANAGEMENT
edited by P. S. Thomas.
Lippincott–Raven Publishers, Philadelphia © 1997

11

Nerve Root Blocks

Jeffrey S. Wang and P. Sebastian Thomas

*Department of Anesthesiology, SUNY Health Science Center at Syracuse,
Syracuse, New York 13210*

ANATOMY

There are 31 pairs of nerve roots which include 8 cervical pairs, 12 thoracic pairs, 5 lumbar pairs, 5 sacral pairs, and 1 coccygeal pair. Cervical roots one through seven emerge from the more cephalad interspace (i.e., cervical root six will emerge from the C5/6 interspace). All other roots will emerge from the more caudad interspace (i.e., cervical root eight, thoracic root six, lumbar root four, and sacral root two will emerge from the C7/T1, T6/7, L4/5, and S2/3 interspaces, respectively (1–4).

Dorsal and ventral root filaments combine to form the spinal ganglion which is covered with a dural sleeve from which the spinal nerves emerge. The nerve roots emerge between the vertebral body and the superior articular surface of the inferior vertebra via the intervertebral foramina.

INDICATIONS

Nerve root blocks may be used if there is symptomatology involving a specific dermatomal pattern. The blocks may be diagnostic, therapeutic, or used for acute pain. Diagnostic blocks are used to help identify the level of the spine where nerve root compression is and which of the nerve roots causes the patient's pain. Nerve root blocks have also been used for chronic pain involving irritation due to neuroforaminal narrowing and/or compression. Thoracic nerve roots have been blocked for injuries such as thoracotomy, fractured ribs, and post herpetic neuralgia.

POSITION

The patient is placed in the prone position on the x-ray table with a pillow under the chest to facilitate flexion of the cervical and thoracic spine, or a pillow under the abdomen to help flex the lumbar spine (Fig. 1). An AP view is obtained after a marker is placed to confirm the correct level for the block.

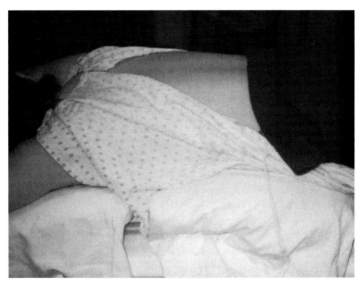

FIG. 1. Patient in prone position on the x-ray table.

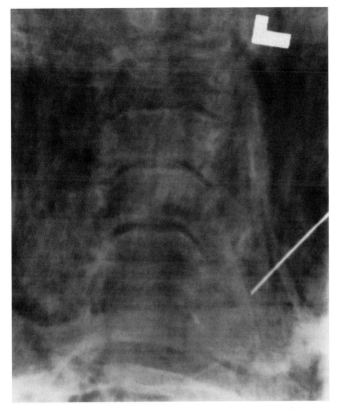

FIG. 2. PA view showing needle in the cervical neuroforamen.

PROCEDURE

Cervical and Thoracic Nerve Roots

After the correct level has been identified and prepped in a sterile fashion with a solution such as betadine, a skin wheal with local anesthetic is placed over the lateral edge of the vertebral body cephalad to the transverse process that is 2 to 4 cm lateral to the midline. A 22-gauge spinal needle is placed straight down until a paresthesia is obtained or bone is contacted (Fig. 2). A lateral view is obtained to confirm proper depth in the intervertebral foramina if there is no paresthesia (Fig. 3). After the final position is obtained, aspiration of the needle should be negative for CSF or blood. Figure 4 shows needle in the neuroforamen at the thoracic nerve root.

Lumbar Nerve Roots

After the correct level has been identified and prepped in a sterile fashion with a solution such as betadine, a skin wheal with local anesthetic is placed 5 to 7 cm lateral to the spinous

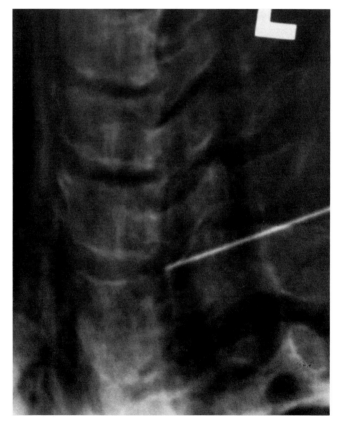

FIG. 3. Lateral view showing needle in the neuroforamen.

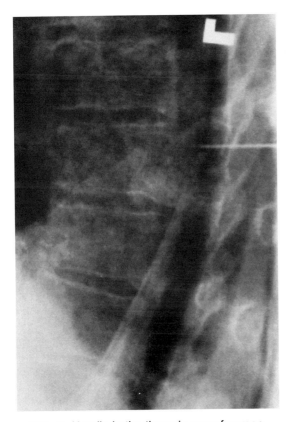

FIG. 4. Needle in the thoracic neuroforamen.

process. A 22-gauge spinal needle is directed at a 45° angle toward the cephalad surface of the transverse process. Another PA view is obtained to confirm lateral position (Fig. 5). If a paresthesia is obtained in the correct dermatomal distribution, an injection should be made.

A lateral view is obtained for final position in the intervertebral foramina if no paresthesia is elicited (Figs. 6A and 6B). After the final position is obtained, aspiration of the needle should be negative for CSF or blood. For lumbar root five, the iliac crest may interfere with lateral positioning of the needle and the procedure for cervical and thoracic nerve root blocks should be followed.

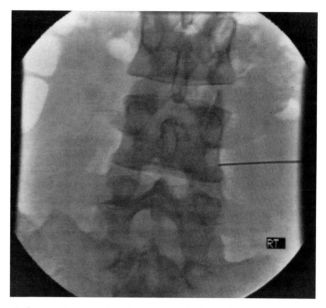

FIG. 5. PA view showing needle in the L4 neuroforamen.

Sacral Nerve Roots

After the correct level has been identified and prepped in a sterile fashion with a solution such as betadine, a skin wheal with local anesthetic is placed over the correct space. A 22-gauge spinal needle should be inserted to the "fish eye" or sacral foramina shown on a PA view (Fig 7). If a paresthesia is obtained in the correct dermatomal distribution, an injection should be made. After the final position is obtained, aspiration of the needle should be negative for CSF or blood. Figure 8 shows needle position in the sacral neuroforamen in a cadaver.

AGENTS

Lidocaine 2% or bupivacaine 0.25–0.5% 2 to 4 cc with methylprednisolone acetate 40 to 80 mg may then be injected.

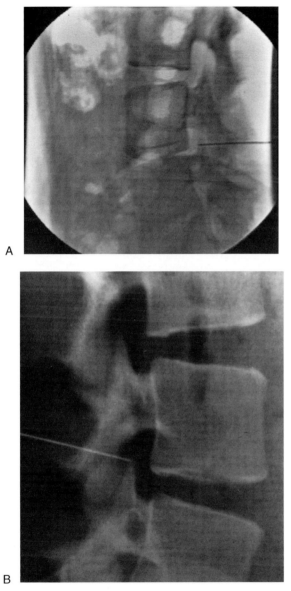

FIG. 6. A: Lateral view showing needle at the tip of the neurofora-men. **B:** Lateral view showing needle inside L4 neuroforamen.

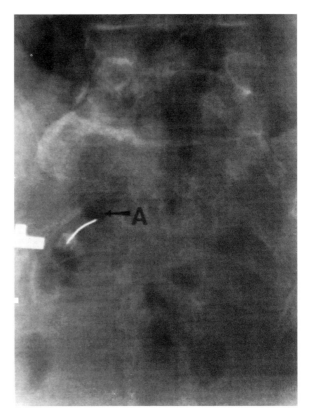

FIG. 7. Needle in sacral neuroforamen "fish eye" is marked (**A**).

COMPLICATIONS

Since there is the presence of a dural cuff at the nerve root, an epidural or subarachnoid injection may occur. With the small volume used, this is usually not a catastrophic problem. An intraneuronal injection may damage the nerve root, so discontinue the injection if it produces pain or has excessive resistance.

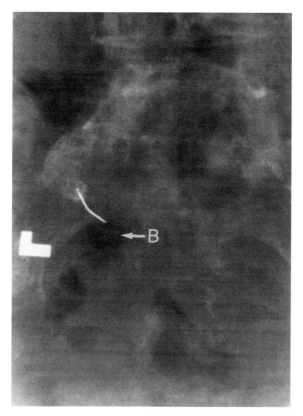

FIG. 8. Needle in the sacral neuroforamen in a cadaver. "Fish eye" is marked (**B**).

REFERENCES

1. Brown DL. *Atlas of regional anesthesia.* WB Saunders, Philadelphia; 1992.
2. Gray H. *Anatomy, descriptive and surgical, 15th ed.* Bounty Books, New York; 1977.
3. Raj PP. *Practical management of pain, 2nd ed.* Mosby Year Book, St Louis; 1992.
4. Urban & Scwartzenberg, Baltimore; 1987.

IMAGE-GUIDED PAIN MANAGEMENT
edited by P. S. Thomas.
Lippincott–Raven Publishers, Philadelphia © 1997

12

Computed Tomography-Guided Celiac Plexus Block

Jeffrey S. Wang and P. Sebastian Thomas

Department of Anesthesiology, SUNY Health Science Center at Syracuse, Syracuse, New York 13210

ANATOMY

The celiac plexus is the largest of the three great plexuses of the sympathetic nervous system, and it innervates the abdominal organs: abdominal viscera, stomach, small bowel, large bowel to the splenic flexure, omentum, liver, biliary tract, pancreas, spleen, adrenal glands, and the kidneys. It is made up of one to five ganglia that range in size from 0.5 to 4.5 cm in diameter. Innervation is derived from T5 to T12 via the greater, lesser, and least splanchnic nerves. The celiac plexus is located anterolateral to the celiac artery and it lays anterior to the aorta (3,6,10). Celiac plexus can be approached in many different ways. Posterior, anterior, and retrocrural are the common approaches. This chapter discusses the posterior approach to the celiac plexus block.

INDICATIONS

Celiac plexus block (CPB) has been used for acute and chronic pain that involves any of the abdominal viscera including such conditions as hepatic arterial embolization, pancreatic carcinoma, chronic pancreatitis, gastric carcinoma (1,2,5,9,15,

16,17,20,21). Blockade for malignancy has been performed using neurolytic agents. A diagnostic block using local anesthetics to determine efficacy should precede any neurolytic blocks of the celiac plexus.

Chronic benign abdominal pain has been treated by some with varying success rates. Long-lasting relief after celiac plexus blocks have not been consistent. Some patients may derive benefit from even a short period of pain relief. The addition of steroids to the injectate may help those patients with an inflammatory process at the plexus. A celiac plexus block may also be used to provide surgical anesthesia for procedures of the biliary tract and abdomen in conjunction with intercostal blocks.

POSITION

The patient is placed in the prone position with a pillow under the abdomen to help flex the lumbar spine (Fig. 1).

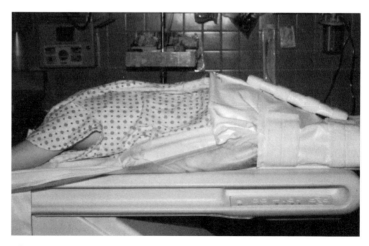

FIG. 1. The patient is placed prone on the CT scanner with a pillow under the abdomen.

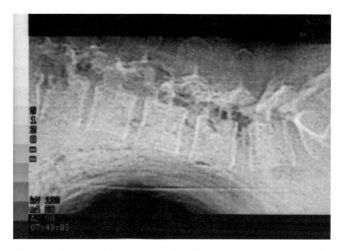

FIG. 2. Lateral scout view showing the lumbar vertebral bodies.

IDENTIFICATION OF LANDMARKS

A lateral scout film is obtained to identify the body of L1 (Fig. 2). Axial sections are obtained at the level of L1, 0.5 cm cephalad, and 0.5 cm caudad, which were made at the level marked by the CT scanner (Fig. 3A). After the axial view is obtained, measurements from the scanner's midline to the needle insertion point, the depth from the needle insertion point to the anterior portion of the vertebral body, and the angle between these lines can be made (Figs. 3B and Fig. 3C).

The CT scanner will project external position marks via laser, which denotes the CT scanner's midline and the level of the chosen transverse section (Fig. 4). This position is marked on the skin with an indelible marker (5,13,14,18).

PROCEDURE

The skin is prepped with an antiseptic solution (betadine) and draped in a sterile fashion. Skin wheals are made with lidocaine 1.0% at the distance from the mark derived from measurement 1.

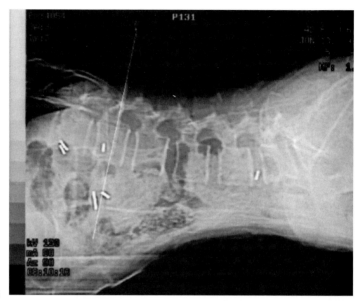

A

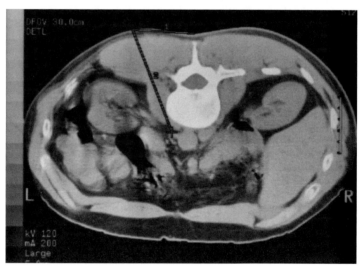

B

FIG. 3. A: Lateral view with the CT scanner's marker over the lower
third of the L1 vertebral body (**B1**). **B:** Axial view at the level depicted
in A. Line 1 is the distance from the scanners midline to the needle
insertion point. Note that the anatomic midline is different from the CT
scanner's midline. Line 2 is the depth from the skin to the anterior portion of the vertebral body. Aorta (*A*), vena cava (*V*), kidneys (*K*), spleen
(*S*) and liver (*L*).

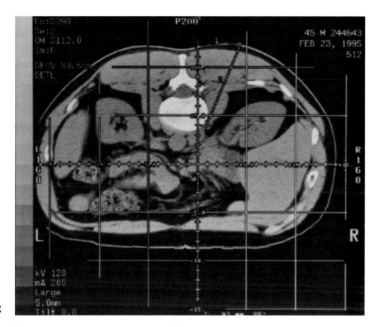

FIG. 3. C: Axial view with the CT scanner's grid overlay to help make the initial measurements.

A 22-gauge 6-inch spinal needle is inserted with an initial angle of 45° to the body of L1, repositioned to the determined angle a to bypass the vertebra, and inserted to the depth determined from measurement 2. A lateral scout film is taken to determine the location of the tip of the needle (Fig. 5).

An axial section is taken at this point to determine the needle tip's final position. After a negative aspiration for blood or CSF, a 2–3 cc test dose is injected. This may include radiopaque contrast dye to confirm spread of the injectate and location of the needle (Fig. 6).

AGENTS

Local anesthetics frequently used for diagnostic blocks include lidocaine 2% and bupivacaine 0.25–0.75%. To perform neurolytic celiac plexus blocks, phenol 6%, or absolute alcohol

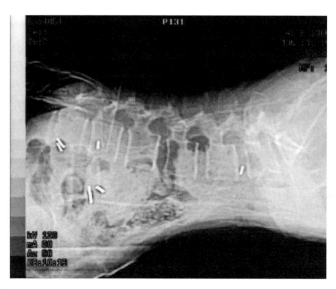

FIG. 4. Lateral scout view showing the needle passing the vertebral body (*B*).

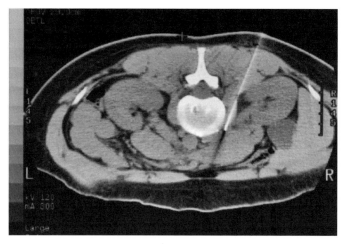

FIG. 5. Axial view showing the tip of the needle *(arrow)* near the vena cava (*V*) for a right-sided celiac plexus block.

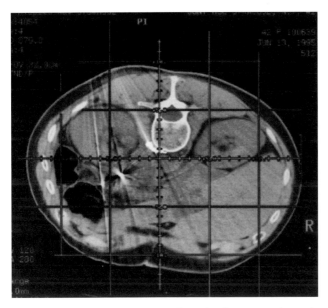

FIG. 6. Axial view with injection of 2 mls of contrast *(arrow)* near the celiac plexus.

is mixed with a volume of local anesthetic to form a 50–100% solution of absolute alcohol. A unilateral block may be performed with a total injected volume of 15 to 20 cc, and a bilateral block may use 30 to 40 cc with half the volume injected through each needle. This volume is smaller than other techniques due to the better accuracy of the CT scanner (4,8,9,15).

COMPLICATIONS

Possible complications that may arise during and after the procedure are due to direct damage as the needle is placed, blockade of the sympathetic nerves, or damage to surrounding structures from the neurolytic agents. These may include but are not limited to: a decrease in blood pressure, pain during and after the injection of the medications, diarrhea, excessive bleeding from puncture of blood vessels, injection into the aorta or inferior vena cava, total spinal paralysis, injury to the kidney, bowel, and sexual dysfunction. There is a small chance that some of these side effects may be permanent.

Alcohol as a neurolytic agent may cause pain during and after the injection. It causes nonselective nervous system tissue damage. The effects may last 4 to 6 months before nerve regeneration occurs (8,20,21).

REFERENCES

1. Bell S, Cole R, Robert-Thompson IC. Celiac plexus block for control of pain in chronic pancreatitis. *Br Med J* 1980;281:1604.
2. Brown DL. A retrospective analysis of neurolytic celiac plexus block for nonpancreatic intra-abdominal cancer pain. *Reg Anesth* 1989;14:63.
3. Brown DL. *Atlas of regional anesthesia.* WB Saunders, Philadelphia, 1992.
4. Brown DL, Bulley TK, Uiel EL. Neurolytic celiac plexus block for pancreatic cancer pain. *Anesth Analg* 1987;66:869–73.
5. Buy JN, Muss AA, Singler RC. CT-guided celiac plexus and splanchnic nerve neurolysis. *J Comput Assist Tomogr* 1982;6:315–319.
6. Clemente CD. *Anatomy: A regional atlas of the human body, 3rd ed.* Urban & Scwartzenberg, Baltimore; 1987.
7. Filshie J, Golding S, Robbie DS, et al. Unilateral computerized tomography guided coeliac plexus block: A technique for pain relief. *Anesthesia* 1983;38:498–503.
8. Galizia EJ, Lahiri SK. Paraplegia following celiac plexus block with phenol. *Br J Anaesth* 1974;46:539–40.
9. Gorbitz C, Leavens ME. Alcohol block of the celiac plexus for control of upper abdominal pain caused by cancer and pancreatitis. *J Neurosurg* 1971;34:575–579.
10. Gray H. *Anatomy, descriptive and surgical, 15th ed.* Bounty Books, New York; 1977.
11. HanKemeier V. Neurolytic celiac plexus block for cancer-related upper abdominal pain using the unilateral puncture technique and lateral position. *Pain* 1987;4:S135.
12. Hegedus V. Relief of pancreatic pain by radiography-guided block. *AJR* 1979;133:1101–1103.
13. Jackson SH, Jacobs JB, Epstein RA. A radiographic approach to celiac plexus block. *Anesthesiol* 1969;31:373–375.
14. Jacobs JB, Jackson SH, Doppman JL. A radiographic approach to celiac ganglion block. *Radiology* 1969;92:1372–1373.
15. Jones J, Gough D. Coeliac plexus block with alcohol for relief of upper abdominal pain due to cancer. *Ann R Coll Surg Engl* 1977;59:46–49.
16. Kune GA, Cole R, Roberts-Thompsin IC. Observations on the relief of pancreatic pain. *Med J Austr* 1975;2:789.

17. Leung JW, Bowen-Wright M, Aveling W, et al. Coeliac plexus block for pain in pancreatic cancer and chronic pancreatitis. *Br J Surg* 1983;70: 730–732.
18. Moore DC, Bush WH, Burnett LL. Celiac plexus block: A roentgeno-graphic, anatomic study of technique and spread of solution in patients and corpses. *Anesth Analg* 1981;60:369–379.
19. Owitz S, Koppolu S. Celiac plexus block: An overview. *Mt Sinai J Med* 1983;50:486–490.
20. Patt RB. *Cancer pain*. JB Lippincott, Philadelphia; 1993.
21. Raj PP. *Practical management of pain, 2nd ed.* Mosby Year Book, St Louis; 1992.

IMAGE-GUIDED PAIN MANAGEMENT
edited by P. S. Thomas.
Lippincott–Raven Publishers, Philadelphia © 1997

13

Radiologically Guided Lumbar Sympathetic Blocks

David G. Fellows

*Department of Anesthesiology, SUNY Health Science Center at Syracuse,
Syracuse, New York 13210*

INDICATIONS

Sympathetic blockade to the lower extremity is most commonly utilized for the treatment and diagnosis of sympathetically mediated pain syndromes. The procedure is also used in attempts to increase blood flow and reduce pain in the treatment of painful peripheral vascular disease and ischemic ulcerations and phantom limb pain.

ANATOMY

The bilateral lumbar sympathetic chains lie in the retroperitoneal space anterolateral to the vertebral bodies and medial to the psoas muscle and the lumbar somatic nerve plexus (3). The genitofemoral nerve courses over the psoas muscle lateral to the sympathetic chain (1). The great vessels lie anteromedial to the chains, with the vena cava being more closely approximated to the right chain than the aorta to the left chain. The kidneys and ureters occupy a posterolateral position to the chains.

PROCEDURE

A clinician's goal in performing a lumbar sympathetic block is to place a needle as close to the chain as possible, while avoiding placing the needle in potentially dangerous areas. Structures to be avoided include the lumbar somatic plexus, the great vessels, the spinal canal, the intervertebral disks, and the renal system. Following placement of an intravenous line, the patient is placed prone on the fluoroscopy table. A pillow is placed under the abdomen to lessen the lumbar lordosis. Following sterile prep and drape, the L2 vertebral spinous process is located by palpation and marked by placing a needle on the overlying skin. The location is confirmed with AP fluoroscopic views by counting down from T12 or by counting up from the sacrum (Figs. 1A and 1B).

At a distance of 10 cm lateral to the L2 spinous process, a skin wheal is made with local anesthesia. A 6-inch 22-gauge spinal needle is then gently advanced at an angle so as to touch the L2 vertebral body. The needle position is confirmed by AP fluoroscopy (Fig. 2). Umeda (4) discovered that the best needle placement for this procedure is at the lower one-third of the body of L2 or the upper one-third of the body of L3. Such placement gives the best chance of hitting the sympathetic ganglia while avoiding the disc space and the lumbar radicular arteries which tend to course over the middle one-third of the vertebral bodies (4).

The depth of the needle is noted and it is withdrawn to the skin. The angle of the needle is then adjusted so as to just miss the vertebral body on the next advancement. This angle is usually close to 45°. Traditionally, the needle is advanced 1 cm deeper than the initial placement.

With x-ray assistance on lateral views, it is easier to advance the needle until it is just at the anterior rim of the vertebral body. Now on an AP view, the needle tip should be seen to have the lateral portion of the vertebral body superimposed on it. This final AP view is essential to avoid a lateral placement of the needle tip in the psoas muscle or even in the kidney.

Cherry and Rao (1) stressed the importance of the initial needle insertion site to avoid needle placement in the psoas muscle and the lumbar somatic nerves. An initial insertion site too close to the midline can require a very steep angle to bypass the vertebral body and will result in a lateral needle tip place-

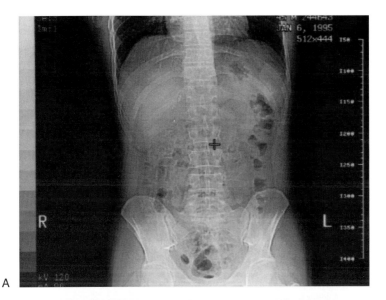

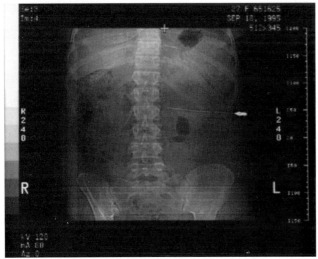

FIG. 1. AP view showing vertebral bodies (**A,B**).

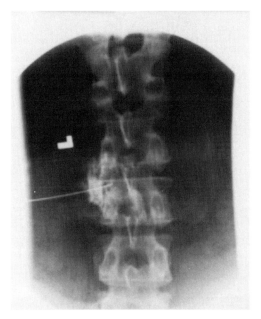

FIG. 2. AP view showing needle position.

ment. They recommend an insertion site for thin patients at 7.5 cm lateral to the spinous process, 10 cm lateral for normal-sized patients, and 12.5 cm lateral for obese patients (1).

Needle position and the spread of local anesthesia can be confirmed by the injection of contrast material (Figs. 3A and 3B). Following negative aspiration of the needle, a mixture of contrast and an appropriate test dose of local anesthesia with epinephrine is injected. On AP views, the contrast should appear to be centered over the lateral portion of the vertebral body (Fig. 3A). No contrast should be seen to fan out in the psoas muscle. On lateral views, the contrast should appear to lie just anterior to the vertebral body (Fig. 3B). There should be very little resistance felt while injecting. Following this, a total of 10 mls of 0.25% bupivacaine is injected, 2 mls at a time, with repeated aspiration of the needle. Hatangdi and Boas (2) showed that 8 to 12 mls of local anesthesia would spread over 2 to 3 vertebral bodies and would virtually ensure

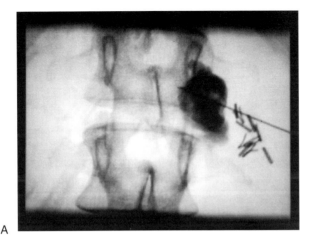

A

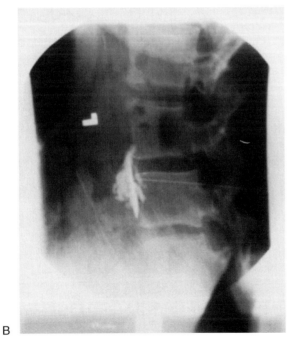

B

FIG. 3. A: AP view showing needle position with contrast material.
B: Lateral view showing needle position with contrast material.

complete sympathetic block (2). They also showed that there is no advantage in blocking the chain at two or more sites over the one needle technique just described.

CASE REPORT 1: X-RAY GUIDED LUMBAR SYMPATHETIC BLOCK

A 27-year-old male injured his left knee at work 2 years prior to presentation to the pain clinic. Nine months earlier, the patient had undergone arthroscopy of his left knee and carried a diagnosis of patellar chondromalacia. The patient complained of burning sensations in his knee and difficult rehabilitation with decreased mobility despite repeated attempts at physical therapy.

Multiple nonsteroid anti-inflammatory agents did not help the patient. On examination, vital signs were unremarkable as was the cardiopulmonary system. Reflexes were intact. Exam of the knee showed no edema and no color or temperature changes. The patient did complain of pain during light touch of the prepatellar area. The remainder of sensory exam was normal. Flexion of the knee was limited to 25%. Motor exam was limited by the patient's pain.

To rule out a sympathetic component to the patient's pain, a diagnostic lumbar paravertebral block was performed. Ten cc of 0.25 marcaine was injected as described in the procedure.

The patient reported 80% relief of his pain for 8 hours, followed by return of some pain to 50% of pre-block levels. A series of sympathetic blocks resulted in overall 60% to 70% reduction of the patient's pain.

CASE REPORT 2: CT-GUIDED LUMBAR SYMPATHETIC BLOCK

Under usual circumstances, the benefits of CT assistance does not seem to justify its added cost. An exception to this may be its use in performing the block on obese patients. CT guidance allows easy identification of anatomic structures. The needle course can be identified and plotted with angles and depth of insertion calculated prior to needle insertion. With CT guidance in obese patients, the chance of renal puncture should be lessened. Another possible use of CT guidance may be for neurolytic block of the sympathetic chain. CT allows pinpoint placement of the needle. The addition of contrast material to the injectate will also allow early identification of any spread toward somatic nerves and further injection could be halted.

The patient was a 27-year-old female with a diagnosis of reflex sympathetic dystrophy. She had injured her leg in a MVA 4 years earlier. Records on initial treatment soon after the trauma indicate the patient had complaints of temperature and color changes and swelling of her leg. The patient complained of persistent pain in her leg. The patient had been treated with a series of repeated lumbar epidural blocks and physical therapy with initial improvement in her symptoms and pain. The patient's pain returned and did not respond as well to epidural blocks and physical therapy. The patient was obese, weighing 110 kg. Her general health, past medical history, and review of symptoms was benign. On exam, her leg was noted to be slightly edematous below the knee. There was a mild hyperesthesia noted. No color changes were observed. No atrophy was noted.

To determine if the patient still had an element of sympathetically mediated pain, a lumbar sympathetic block was decided on. Because of the patient's obesity, CT guidance was used. Following IV placement, the patient was placed prone on the CT table. Her back was prepped and draped. A scout film was obtained. The L2 level was noted and marked (Figs. 1A and 1B). At the L2 level, a cross-sectional scan was taken (Fig. 4). A needle course was then plotted so as to correctly place the needle, while missing other vital structures. The CT technician calculated the distance from the midline for the entry point of the needle. The angle of insertion and depth of insertion was also calculated (Fig. 5). Local anesthesia was injected at the projected skin entry point and a 6-inch spinal needle advanced as plotted. Following confirmation of correct placement by CT verification, 1 cc of radio opaque dye (Omnipac 180) was

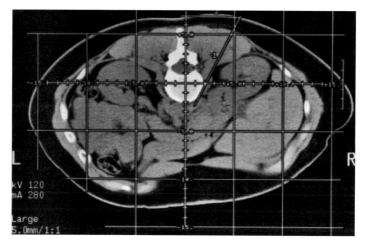

FIG. 4. Cross-sectional scan with grid showing via line two the distance from midline to point of entry and by line 1 the angle and approximate depth of needle.

injected to document the spread (Fig. 6). A total of 10 mls of 0.25% bupivacaine was injected slowly with multiple negative aspirations.

The patient's leg was noted to be warmer and the patient reported 8 hours of improvement in her pain. Her pain did

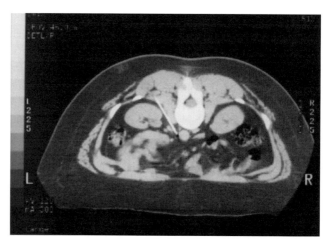

FIG. 5. Cross-sectional scan showing tip of the needle.

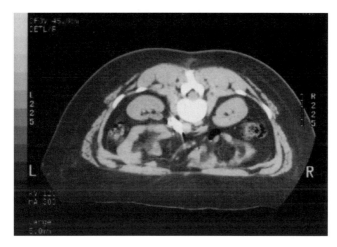

FIG. 6. Cross-sectional scan showing spread of the dye.

return to baseline levels. Further sympathetic blocks provided only temporary relief of her pain. The patient is currently considering dorsal column stimulation as a treatment for her sympathetically mediated pain.

REFERENCES

1. Cherry DA, Rao OM. Lumbar sympathetic and celiac plexus blocks. *Brit J Anaesthesia* 1982;54:1037–1039.
2. Hatangdi VS, Boas RA. Lumbar sympathectomy: A single needle technique. *Brit J Anaesthesia* 1985;57:285–289.
3. Raj PP, ed. *Practical management of pain, 2nd ed.* Mosby Year Book, St. Louis; 1992.
4. Umeda, et al. Cadaver anatomic analysis of the best site for chemical lumbar sympathectomy. *Anes Analg* 1987;66:643–646.

IMAGE-GUIDED PAIN MANAGEMENT
edited by P. S. Thomas.
Lippincott–Raven Publishers, Philadelphia © 1997

14

Epidural Neurolytic Block

Andrew M. Sopchak

Department of Radiology, University of Buffalo,
Buffalo, New York 14214

OVERVIEW

Neurolytic blockade has the potential for the clinician in pain management of providing pain relief to those patients with severe and intractable pain. These patients most frequently have pain caused by advanced cancer. Other incurable diseases such as occlusive vascular disease may also be amenable to this modality of treatment (1,3).

PATIENT CONSIDERATIONS

Prior to consideration of any patient for neurolytic blockade, a complete pain management plan must be formulated. This plan must take into consideration the patient's history, especially focusing on the cause of their pain, treatments performed, and any ongoing social factors. Most, if not all, patients considered for neurolytic blockade have been treated for some period of time with opioid analgesics. When satisfactory pain control is no longer obtained with oral analgesics or the side effects become intolerable, then it is reasonable to consider neurolytic blockade. However, it is important to remember that despite successful neurolytic blockade, many patients will continue to require some level of oral analgesics. A long history of analgesic use causing tolerance combined with the

107

spread of the primary disease process beyond the anatomic limits of the neurolytic block being performed, almost guarantee that oral analgesic supplementation will be required.

PATIENT SELECTION

There are important differences that must be considered when choosing the epidural neurolytic block. The block produced by the epidural neurolytic block is bilateral and more diffuse, when compared with a subarachnoid neurolytic block with which one can produce a focalized unilateral segmental blockade. As a result of its more diffuse spread, neurologic complications are more common, especially in the sacral area.

It is important, as with any procedure, to discuss the risks and benefits of the procedure chosen. Any patient who is hesitant or frankly uncooperative will be a poor candidate for neurolytic blockade. It is also essential that prior to any neurolytic block, a reversible diagnostic block be performed with local anesthetic in order to better determine whether the patient is a suitable candidate for the neurolytic procedure.

Of those neurolytic agents or techniques available, the two in most common clinical use are ethyl alcohol and phenol. Probably secondary to its local anesthetic properties, phenol causes little pain on injection. However, CNS and cardiovascular toxic side effects, although rare in the doses used clinically, can occur. The only significant side effect of ethyl alcohol injection is pain on injection. Local anesthetic prior to ethanol injection can reduce the pain; however, it can make identifying and verifying proper placement of the block more difficult.

The epidural neurolytic block is often selected when the site of pain is above the T6 level. The shape and capacity of the spinal canal above T6 makes it difficult to achieve consistent results.

Prior to performing the block the patient should have an MRI to evaluate tumor invasion in the area of the block. Tumor invasion in the area may make the block too unpredictable, and the increased risk of bleeding which can result in cord compression may make the risks of the procedure outweigh the benefits.

TECHNIQUE

The procedure is started with the placement of an epidural catheter at or near the level of block desired. Because we are going to be doing a neurolytic block, the effects of which will last a long time, it is imperative that precise catheter placement be verified. This should be done with injection of a small amount of contrast media. This will produce a diffuse outline anterior to the posterior wall of the vertebral canal. AP view and a lateral view will confirm the position and the spread of the dye as shown in Figures 1 and 2. This is in contrast to subarachnoid and subdural injection. The catheter position can also be verified by injection of small doses of local anesthetics, such as 2 ml of 1% lidocaine at 15-minute intervals ideally producing a narrow segmental band of sensory loss. This can be distinguished from a subdural block which would be diffuse and patchy and a subarachnoid block which would be much wider in area and solid.

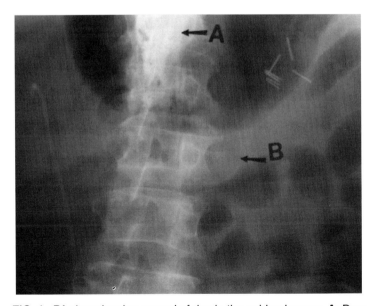

FIG. 1. PA view showing spread of dye in the epidural space. **A**: Dye; **B**: Epidural catheter.

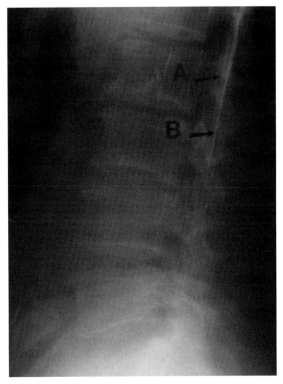

FIG. 2. Lateral view showing spread of dye in the epidural space. **A**: Dye; **B**: Epidural catheter.

Once confirmation of catheter placement is achieved, at least 2 hours must elapse from the time of lidocaine administration for the block to wear off. This is extremely important as residual blockade may cause the neurolytic agent to spread further than expected and result in a wider area of neurolysis than had been anticipated.

Several different authors have used various different modifications of this basic technique. Racz et al. (6) used 5.5% phenol in saline after confirmation of the catheter position by radiography, aspiration, and injection of 3 ml of 0.5% bupivacaine (6). After waiting 24 hours of placement, they used 2.5 to 5 ml in the cervical region. They report the use of this technique in cancer pain, reflex sympathetic dystrophy, and chronic pain syndromes with spasticity.

Colpitts et al. (2) placed the epidural in the usual fashion with its tips in the center of the band of pain and 3 to 4 ml of 1–2% lidocaine was injected to determine the proper volume of phenol required to relieve the pain (4). Pain relief varied from 3 weeks to 4.5 months.

Korevaar (5) also placed the epidural catheter so its tip is in the center of the dermatomal pain distribution (5). He used 5 to 7 ml of 0.25% bupivacaine to evaluate for correct catheter placement.

He then injected increments of 0.2 ml of absolute alcohol until 3 to 5 ml had been injected over 20 to 30 minutes. Second and third daily injections were performed unless the patients had 100% relief.

Post-injection patients were followed closely and 89% were considered to have been treated successfully with a 70% or greater pain relief with at least 25% decrease in narcotic usage.

Dobrogowski et al. (4) reported on the treatment of 44 patients with cancer pain. After the epidural was placed in the standard manner, 4 to 6 ml of 1% lidocaine was injected to locate the correct spinal segments and to obtain a close estimate on the volume required for neurolytic block.

After the pain reappeared, a 6% aqueous phenol solution was injected. In 26 patients the injection was repeated from 7 days to 5 months after the first administration. The average duration of pain relief was 38 days. There were no toxic side effects such as urinary retention found in the study.

REFERENCES

1. Bonica JJ. *The management of pain, 2nd ed.* Lea & Febiger, Philadelphia; 1990.
2. Colpitts MR, Levy DA, Lawrence M. *Treatment of cancer related pain with phenol epidural block* [Abstract]. Presented at the Second World Congress on Pain, Montreal; 1978.
3. Cousins MJ, Bridenbaugh PO. *Neural blockade in clinical anesthesia and management of pain, 2nd ed.* JB Lippincott, Philadelphia; 1988.

4. Dobrogowski J, Kus M. Epidural neurolytic block in cancer patients. In: Erdman, Oyama, Pernak, eds. *The pain clinic I.* Proceedings of the First International Symposium. VNU Science Press, Utrecht, The Netherlands; 1985:51–54.

5. Korevaar WC. Transcatheter thoracic epidural neurolysis using ethyl alcohol. *Anesth* 1988;69:989.

6. Racz GB, Heavner J, Haynsworth P. Repeat epidural phenol injections in chronic pain and spasticity. In: S. Lipton, ed. *Persistent pain: Modern methods of treatment.* Grune & Stratton, New York; 1977;5:61–99.

IMAGE-GUIDED PAIN MANAGEMENT
edited by P. S. Thomas.
Lippincott–Raven Publishers, Philadelphia © 1997

15

Computed Tomography-Guided Hypogastric Plexus Block

Jeffrey S. Wang and P. Sebastian Thomas

Department of Anesthesiology, SUNY Health Science Center at Syracuse, Syracuse, New York 13210

ANATOMY

The hypogastric plexus provides sympathetic innervation to the visceral organs of the pelvis. The plexus is located anterior to the superior border of the sacrum between the common iliac arteries. It is formed from fibers from the lumbar sympathetic ganglion and aortic plexuses. There are no discreet ganglia at this area (1,2,4,7).

INDICATIONS

Patients who have pelvic pain which has been refractory to other conventional treatments including epidural or caudal blocks are candidates for hypogastric plexus blocks. The common indications include pelvic cancer pain and selected cases of interstitial cystitis (5–12).

POSITION

The patient is placed in the prone position with one or two pillows under the lower abdomen to help flex the lumbar spine.

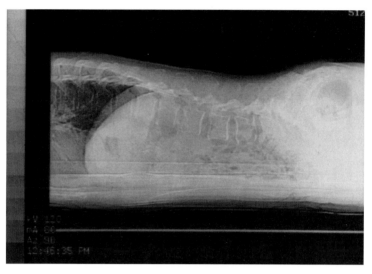

FIG. 1. Lateral scout view showing the lumbar and sacral vertebral bodies.

IDENTIFICATION OF LANDMARKS

A lateral scout film is obtained to identify the body of L5 and/or S1. Transverse sections are obtained from the scout film at the level of L5, 0.5 cm cephalad, and 0.5 cm caudad (Fig. 1). When the lower third of the body of L5 is identified, measurements 1, 2, and angle *a* are obtained (Figs. 2A and 2B).

The CT scanner will project external position marks via laser (Fig. 3) which denotes the CT scanner's midline and the level of the chosen transverse section (Fig. 4). This position is marked on the skin with an indelible marker.

PROCEDURE

The skin is prepped with betadine and draped in a sterile fashion. Skin wheals are made with lidocaine 1% at the distance from the mark derived from measurement 1.

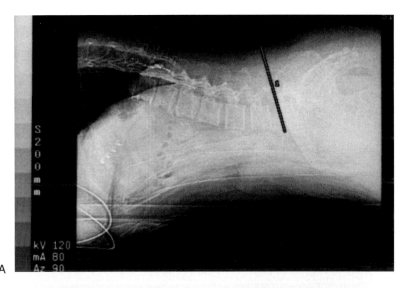

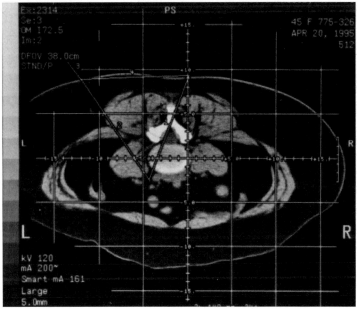

FIG. 2. A: Lateral view with the CT scanner's marker over the lower third of the L5 vertebral body (*B5*). **B:** Axial view at the level of the L5 vertebral body showing the psoas muscles (*P*) and the iliac arteries (*I*).

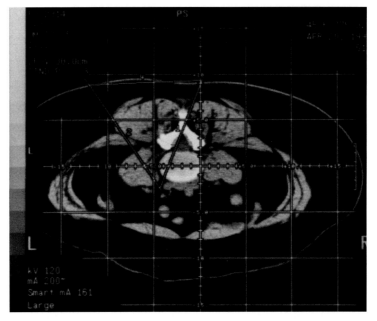

FIG. 3. Axial view with the CT scanner's grid. Line 4 is the distance from the scanner's midline to the needle insertion point. Note that the anatomic midline is different from the CT scanner's midline. Line 2 is the depth from the skin to the anterior portion of the vertebral body.

A 22-gauge 6-inch spinal needle is inserted with an initial angle of 45° to the body of L5 or S1, repositioned to the determined angle *a* to bypass the vertebra, and inserted to the depth determined from measurement 2. A lateral scout film is taken to determine the location of the tip of the needle (Figs. 5 and 6).

A transverse section is now taken to determine the needle tip's final position. The needle should rest at the lower third of the body of L5 and all S1 (Fig. 7). After a negative aspiration for blood or CSF, a 2 cc–3 cc test dose is injected. This may include radiopaque contrast dye to confirm spread of the injectate and location of the needle (Fig. 8).

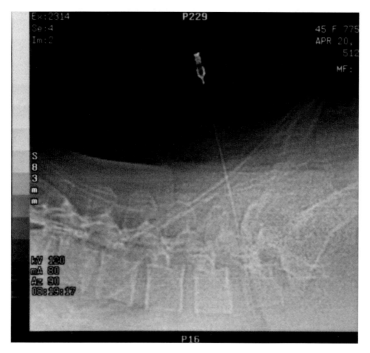

FIG. 4. Lateral scout view showing the needle passing the vertebral body (**B5**).

AGENTS

Local anesthetics frequently used for diagnostic blocks include lidocaine 2% and bupivacaine 0.25–0.75%. To perform neurolytic celiac plexus blocks, phenol 6% or absolute alcohol is mixed with an equal volume of local anesthetic. A unilateral block may be performed with a total injected volume of 10 to 15 cc, and a bilateral block may use 20 to 30 cc with half the volume injected through each needle.

COMPLICATIONS

Possible complications that may arise during and after the procedure include but are not limited to: intra-arterial injection

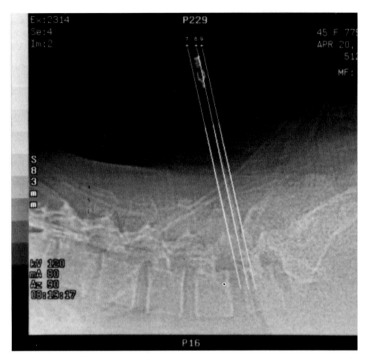

FIG. 5. Lateral scout film with the CT scanner's marker for the axial cut. Note the hub of the needle.

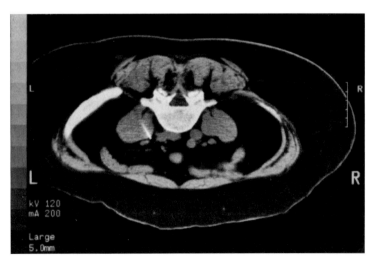

FIG. 6. Axial view showing the tip of the needle in the psoas muscle *(P)*.

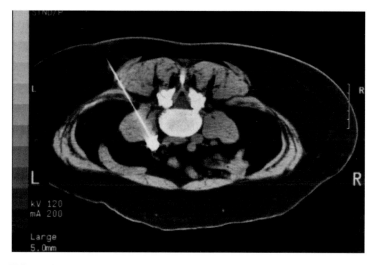

FIG. 7. Axial view with injection of 2 mls of contrast near the hypogastric plexus.

into a blood vessel (aorta or iliac arteries or the vena cava or iliac veins), pain during and after injection of the medications, excessive bleeding, infection, total spinal paralysis, bowel, bladder, or sexual dysfunction. There is a small chance that some of these complications may be permanent.

Alcohol as a neurolytic agent may cause pain during and after the injection. It causes nonselective nervous system tissue damage. The effects may last 4 to 6 months before nerve regeneration occurs.

REFERENCES

1. Brown DL. *Atlas of regional anesthesia.* WB Saunders, Philadelphia; 1992.
2. Clemente CD. *Anatomy: A regional atlas of the human body, 3rd ed.* Urban & Scwartzenberg, Baltimore; 1987.
3. Frier A. Pelvic neurectomy in gynecology. *Obstet Gynecol* 1965; 25:48.
4. Gray H. *Anatomy: Descriptive and surgical, 15th ed.* Bounty Books, New York; 1977.
5. Kent E, deLeon-Cassasota OA, Lema M. Neurolytic superior hypogastric plexus block for cancer related pelvic pain. *Pain* 1992;17(Suppl):19.

6. Lee RB, Stone K, Magelssen, et al. Presacral neurotomy for chronic pelvic pain. *Obstet Gynecol* 1986;68:517.
7. Patt RB. *Cancer pain.* JB Lippincott, Philadelphia; 1993.
8. Plancarte R, et al. Hypogastric plexus block: Retroperitoneal approach. *Anesthesiology* [Absract]. 1989;71:739.
9. Plancarte R, Amescua C, Patt R, et al. Superior hypogastric plexus block for pelvic pain. *Anesthesiology* 1990;73:236.
10. Raj PP. *Practical management of pain, 2nd ed.* Mosby Year Book, St Louis; 1992.
11. Renaer M. *Chronic pelvic pain in women.* Springer-Verlag, New York; 1981.
12. Waldman SD, Wilson WL, Kreps RD. Superior hypogastric plexus block using a single needle and computed tomography guidance: Description of a modified technique. *Regional Anesthesia* 1991;16:286.

IMAGE-GUIDED PAIN MANAGEMENT
edited by P. S. Thomas.
Lippincott–Raven Publishers, Philadelphia © 1997

16

Sacral Nerve Root Block

Syed I. Hosain and P. Sebastian Thomas

Department of Anesthesiology, SUNY Health Science Center at Syracuse, Syracuse, New York 13210

INDICATIONS

The sacral plexus is the parasympathetic nerve supply of the pelvic viscera. The bladder, bowel, and sphincters of the rectum are innervated by the pudendal nerve formed from the sacral nerves. Blockade of the sacral nerves can be utilized to provide relief of pain due to injury of the sacral nerve roots, and is also combined with lumber paravertebral block to produce complete anesthesia of the lower extremity. It also represents a means of blocking the sciatic nerve very early in its origin. Sacral nerve root block can be used both diagnostically and therapeutically for patients with sacral nerve root neuropathies.

ANATOMY

The anterior divisions of the first three sacral nerves and the fourth and fifth lumber nerves form the sacral plexus. The nerves of the sacral plexus divide into two sets, the *terminal* and the *collateral* nerves. The collateral branches supply the pudendal plexus, gluteal structures, the hip joint, and the adductor muscles. The terminal branches supply the sciatic nerve. The anterior sacral nerves S2, S3, S4 form the parasympathetic nerve supply to the pelvic viscera.

121

The sacral nerves exit from the sacrum. The sacrum is a wedge shaped bone made up of the fused lower five vertebrae. On the posterior surface are two rows of openings—the posterior sacral foramina present on each side of the fused spinous processes. Posteriorly, the divisions of the sacral nerves pass through these openings. The posterior sacral foramina are in relation to the corresponding anterior sacral foramina. These posterior foramina are angled slightly medially. The depth of the sacral canal (from posterior sacral foramen to anterior sacral foramen) varies from 2.5 cm at the cephalad end of the sacrum, to 0.5 cm at the caudad end of the sacrum. The difference in the depth of the sacral canal is critical to conduct of a trans sacral nerve root block. The anterior relations of the sacrum are to the pelvic organs, the rectum, bladder, uterus, sympathetic plexus, and vessels of the pelvis (1).

TECHNIQUE OF THE BLOCK

During the conduct of this block the patient is placed in a prone position with a pillow under the hips. The surface anatomy of the first sacral canal is a point 1 cm medial and 1 cm below the posterior superior iliac spine. This position is marked with a marking needle (Fig. 1). The fourth sacral canal is identified at a point 0.5 cm cephalad and just lateral to the sacral cornu of the side to be blocked. This position is marked on the skin surface. Then a line is drawn to connect these two points. The midpoint of this line is the surface landmark of the third sacral foramen. The line is extended cephalad and at a point 1 to 2 cm cephalad to the marker of the second sacral foramen a marker is placed. This will lie approximately opposite the posterior superior iliac spine (2). Then an anteroposterior fluoroscopic image of the area (the sacral foramina) is obtained. The foramina are identified as "fish eyes" on this view (Fig. 2).

An 8 to 10 cm 22-gauge needle is required to reach the first and second sacral foramina. A shorter needle may be employed at the lower sacral foramina. This is due to the presence of more soft tissue at the cephalad end of the sacrum than at the

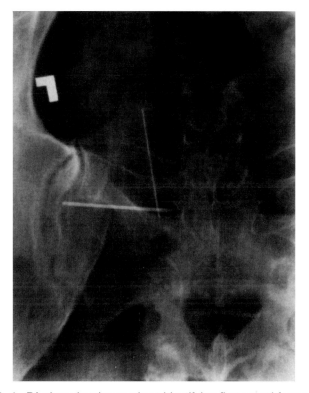

FIG. 1. PA view showing markers identifying first sacral foramen.

caudad end. The needles are directed to touch the bone adjacent to the foramina.

The needles are then walked into the sacral canal in a medial direction. The use of fluoroscopy will aid this process by defining the position of the needle in relation to the foramina.

The needle is advanced into the first sacral canal to a depth of 2.5 cm. The needles are inserted in a descending pattern from S2 to S4. Recalling the decrease in the depth of the subsequent foramina, the needles should be advanced to a slightly lesser depth at each level, in decrements of 0.5 cm. Once the needles are in place, a volume of 7 cc of local anesthetic can be injected into the first sacral canal. Each subsequent injection should be reduced by a volume of 1 cc. The last injection being

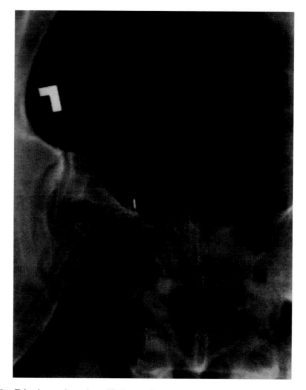

FIG. 2. PA view showing "fish eye" and the needle in the sacral foramen.

made at S4 level with a volume of 3 cc. Our practice is to use 0.25% bupivacaine with methylprednisolone.

COMPLICATIONS AND SIDE EFFECTS

In principle this block may produce loss of parasympathetic function in the bladder and rectal sphincter; however, these are infrequently seen unless a bilateral block is performed. Sympathetic block and the associated hypotension are uncommon unless large volumes of local anesthetic are injected. If the block needles are inserted beyond the recommended depths the pelvic organs are in danger of being damaged. Contamination of the sacral canal contents with fecal material may occur as the needle is withdrawn. In rare instances, the dural sac which is said to end at the lower border of the S2 vertebral body may be punctured due to individual variations in anatomy.

REFERENCES

1. The sacrum, osteology. In: Warwick R, Williams PL, eds. *Gray's anatomy, 35th ed.* Longman Group, Edinburgh; 1978:242–244.
2. Bridenbaugh PO. Sacral plexus nerve block, In: Cousins MJ, Bridenbaugh PO, eds. *The lower extremity: Somatic blockade, neural blockade in clinical anesthesia and management of pain, 2nd ed.* JB Lippincott, Philadelphia; 1988:422–423.

IMAGE-GUIDED PAIN MANAGEMENT
edited by P. S. Thomas.
Lippincott–Raven Publishers, Philadelphia © 1997

17

Posterior Primary Division Nerve Block

Syed I. Hosain and P. Sebastian Thomas

Department of Anesthesiology, SUNY Health Science Center at Syracuse, Syracuse, New York 13210

INDICATIONS

The diagnosis of pain arising from the vertebral column has traditionally been based on morphological changes evident on radiological investigations such as plain radiographs, computerized axial tomography (CAT), and myelography. Recently, the use of magnetic resonance imaging (MRI) has added to the imaging armamentarium. However, these techniques have not been completely successful in defining the pathology or site of the lesion causing the pain. This has prompted the development of newer more physiological-based approaches to the diagnosis of pain syndromes. This approach is illustrated in the case of zygapophyseal joint disease. This condition was given the name *facet joint syndrome* in 1963 by Ghormley (3). Confirmation that certain kinds of back pain arise from disease of the zygapophyseal joints came in the 1970s when Mooney and Robertson reproduced a characteristic dull aching pain in the lower back and lower extremities of volunteer who were previously healthy by stimulation of the zygapophyseal joints (4).

However, although the pain is said to be in the lower back and to radiate to the lower extremities, the precise distribution does not correlate with the segmental level of the joint disease.

ANATOMICAL CONSIDERATIONS

After emerging from the intervertebral foramen, each spinal nerve gives off a meningeal branch and then almost immediately splits into dorsal and anterior divisions. The posterior primary division gives a medial branch that supplies innervation to the zygapophyseal joint. Each joint is formed by the articular processes of two vertebral bodies, one above and one below. The innervation follows a similar pattern; one medial branch is derived from the upper vertebral level and one from the lower (2). The only exception to this rule being the C2–C3 zygapophyseal joint, which the third cervical nerve innervates. The L1 to L4 medial branches form a constant relation to the roots of the lumber transverse processes as follows. The posterior primary division exits between the respective intervertebral foramina. It then crosses the upper border of the lower transverse process running in a groove between the lower transverse process and the superior articular process. Each nerve hooks medially under the mamillo-accessory ligament to cross the lamina of the vertebra. The L5 nerve root follows a constant course over the ala of the sacrum. The C4–C7 medial branches wrap around the waists of the articular pillar of the vertebrae. The C8 medial branch hooks medially onto the lamina of T1. The target area for L1 to L4 zygapophyseal joints is the posterior surface of the most medial end of the transverse process just below its superior border. For the L5 joint the target area is the ala of the sacrum.

TECHNIQUE OF PERFORMING THE BLOCK

The patient is placed in the prone position on the x-ray imaging table. Preparations and facilities must be available to deal with any complications of the block. We employ a wedge to flex the lumber spine. The target area is identified for the block. A 22- or 20-gauge 3 1/2-inch needle is inserted between 3 and 5 cm lateral to the target area. The needle is then guided ventrally and medially toward the target area with repeated fluoroscopy. The needle should rest on the upper medial gutter of the transversal processes (Fig. 1). An oblique view at 45°

and an anteroposterior view at 90° will allow the operator accurately to position the needle in relation to the target area. The tip of the needle should rest on bone and it should not be possible to direct the needle any more medially. The 45° oblique view will demonstrate the classical "Scotty dog" appearance (Fig. 2). The needle should be positioned so that the tip lies on the "eye" of the dog. The outline of the Scotty dog is formed by the articulations of the facet joint and the body of the lower vertebra in oblique view. The needle is withdrawn 1 or 2 mm and then the injection of local anesthetic performed (1). We recommend a volume of 1 to 2 cc of bupivacaine 0.25% or 0.5% or lidocaine 1% with a long acting steroid.

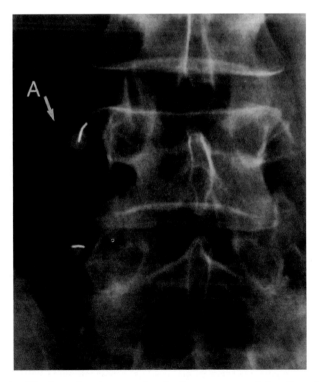

FIG. 1. AP view showing needles in the upper medial gutter of the transverse processes. **A**: Transverse process.

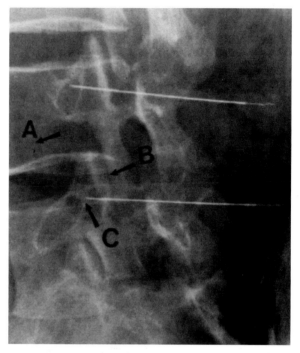

FIG. 2. Oblique (45°) view showing needles on the "eye of the Scotty dog." **A**: Vertebral body; **B**: Facet joint; **C**: "Eye of the Scotty dog."

COMPLICATIONS

These include inadvertent subarachnoid, epidural, intravascular injection. Careful positioning of the needle and aspiration prior to injection will avoid these complications.

REFERENCES

1. Bogduk N. Back pain: Zygapophyseal blocks and epidural steroids. In: Cousins MJ, Bridenbaugh PO, eds. *Neural blockade in clinical anesthesia and management of pain, 2nd ed.* JB Lippincott, Philadelphia; 1988: 935–954.

2. The Joints of the Vertebral Arches in Arthrology. In: Warwick R, Williams PL, eds. *Gray's anatomy, 35th ed.* Longman Group, Edinburgh; 1978:413–414.
3. Ghormley RK. Low back pain with special reference to the articular facet with presentation of an operative procedure. *JAMA* 1963;10:1773.
4. Mooney V, Robertson J. The facet syndrome. *Clin Orthop* 1976;115:149.

IMAGE-GUIDED PAIN MANAGEMENT
edited by P. S. Thomas.
Lippincott–Raven Publishers, Philadelphia © 1997

18

Intra-Articular Facet Block

Thomas D. Masten and Bruce E. Fredrickson

*Department of Orthopedic Surgery, SUNY Health Science Center
at Syracuse, Syracuse, New York 13210*

ZYGAPOPHYSEAL (FACET)
JOINT INJECTIONS

Image-guided spinal pain management by zygapophyseal (facet) joint injection is a controversial area (7). The current state of the art of zygapophyseal (z)-joint injections suggest that these joints are indeed sources of spine pain (8,14,29). Injections of either the z joint or its nerve supply (medial branches) can be valuable in diagnosing which patients have this as a source of pain (3,5,8,14,30,31). Unfortunately, the best therapeutic intervention for this diagnosis is not yet known (8,9,12,17,26).

ANATOMY

The spinal vertebra articulate anteriorly by intervertebral discs and posteriorly by paired joints often called *facet joints*, or more precisely, *zygapophyseal (Z) joints*. Z joints are synovial joints innervated by small articular branches from the medial branches of the posterior dorsal rami arising from the adjacent segmental nerves. Both the synovium as well as the fibrous capsule have nociceptive pain fibers. Z joints are a potential source for spine and extremity pain (11).

PATHOPHYSIOLOGY

Historically, the lumbar spine z joints were initially thought to be the source of pain when they were arthritic, whereas others felt strain of the joint was the source for lumbar pain as well as sciatica (8). Studies by Mooney and others suggested that patients who present with spine pain may well have the z joint as a source for pain (8,14,30).

DIAGNOSIS

History and physical, looking for pathognomonic clinical signs, as well as imaging have been disappointing when tested to clarify the diagnosis of z-joint pain (23,24). Diagnostic injections of the z joint and/or its medial branches seem to be the best way to clarify if that is indeed a patient's source of pain (8,14,26,29).

Clinical signs may be helpful in deciding who may benefit from diagnostic z-joint injections. In the lumbar spine, a typical z-joint clinical profile may include pain aggravated by forward flexion and straight leg raising (23). However, a combination of groin or thigh pain, paraspinal tenderness, and a common test for lumbar z-joint pain provocation with extension rotation when grouped along with abnormal imaging proved to be somewhat specific but not sensitive for z-joint pain when reviewed retrospectively after z-joint blocks. However, they may be predictive of who will most likely get prolonged (more than 6 months) benefit from z-joint blocks with steroid (24).

Noninvasive imaging is not currently considered adequate for diagnosing z-joint pain (31,33). Injection techniques have been used to show that abnormal findings on imaging do not indicate which joints are the source of pain. Some joints that appear to have abnormal imaging (arthroses) may be pain free on pain provocation injections. Joints that appear to be normal may have significant pain elicited on provocation injection followed by pain relief with local anesthetic (8,14). New imaging techniques such as high resolution scanning or pillar views of the C-spine looking for subchondral or articular pillar fractures (1), may also prove to be helpful but are not yet proven. Imaging may still be valuable to rule out anatomic variants, facet orientation, facet anomalies, or pathology (e.g., cysts).

Z-JOINT INJECTIONS, THE TWO BLOCK PARADIGM

Z-joint injections may stimulate a reproduction of a patient's pain due to the noxious irritant effect of saline, radiopaque dye, or local anesthetic. This is suggestive of a diagnosis but not considered proof. If a patient's pain is resolved when the local anesthetic effect has occurred, there is evidence that the z joint is the source of pain. Studies suggest that intra-articular and medial branch blocks are equally effective in diagnosing the z joint as the source of pain (2,5,8). However, Bogduk and others have noted that the placebo effect of z-joint blocks (intra-articular or medial branches) may be as high as 38% (31,32). To control for this, an initial block of the z joint is carried out with local anesthetic (e.g., lidocaine/short acting). If apparent relief of symptoms occur, an additional confirmatory step of blocking the joint on a separate visit using a local anesthetic with a different duration of action (e.g., bupivacaine/long acting) is carried out. (8,14,15,16,32). If the patient again claims relief but the duration of the relief is consistent with the duration of the blocking agent (different, e.g., longer than the first block), this is considered a true positive response.

THERAPEUTIC BENEFIT

The therapeutic benefit of z-joint blocks is less clear and is controversial (12,26). Potential risks and benefits must be weighed. Some will use this as an adjunct to other conservative care [mechanical therapy (e.g., McKenzie techniques), manual techniques, functional restoration including stretching and strengthening, spine stabilization, etc.]. Some term this use as "opening a therapeutic window of opportunity," in which repeated trials of conservative care may show additional benefit (20). If prolonged response cannot be gained with the first injection, then repeating in a series is not encouraged.

The lumbar spine has more support for using intra-articular z-joint injections for therapeutic purposes. Unfortunately, there does not seem to be a clear way to predict who will get long-term benefit.

The cervical spine z-joint blocks have anecdotal evidence for long-term therapeutic benefit in some patients with neck pain. Unfortunately, it is not the majority of patients. Barnsley et al. noted the lack of effect of z-joint injections with corticosteroid for chronic pain following whiplash injury. Less than 50% had benefit more than 1 week and less than 20% had benefit more than 1 month. It was interesting to note that this benefit occurred just as often in those receiving the local anesthetic as those receiving betamethasone (6).

Once the diagnosis of z-joint pain is made, other alternatives to be considered include denervation (9) (e.g., radiofrequency, cryotherapy, or chemical), prolotherapy (21b), or surgery. These are still being evaluated and require further study.

SUMMARY OF INDICATIONS AND CONSIDERATIONS REGARDING Z-JOINT INJECTIONS (17)

Diagnosis

To clarify the source of spine or extremity pain that is not responding to direct conservative therapy for more than the usual time course (approximately 4 weeks or more) typically expected for resolution of pain by natural history. If the z joint is suspected, then injection procedures are indicated.

Therapy

Possible benefit for lumbar spine, less likely for cervical spine, and not clearly studied for thoracic spine.

Importance of Fluoroscopy

Fluoroscopic guidance is indicated for z joint and medial branch blocks. Bi-plane fluoroscopy can be used efficiently, however, a good C-arm is sufficient. Additional time may be taken to observe (e.g., right angle) views prior to injection but this is often required to ensure a safe procedure (especially in the cervical and thoracic area). Contrast medium is recommended as a useful marker to clarify intra-articular injection (3,5,8,15,16). It can also be useful in precision location of medial branch blocks.

Absence of Pathognomonic Findings

There are no clinical findings by history or physical that have been clearly proven to diagnose z-joint pathology (8,30). Consequently, systematically blocking each z joint is indicated as the preferred method of diagnosing the exact location of the source of pain. Some use H & P to try and localize pathology whereas others start with the statistically most common pain sources (31,32,34).

FALSE POSITIVES/PLACEBO EFFECT

The two-block paradigm suggested by Bogduk and others should seriously be considered to minimize the placebo effect (8,14,15,16,32).

CONTRAINDICATIONS

Bleeding Diatheses
Infection
Drug Allergy
Diabetes Mellitus
Artificial Heart Valves, MVP
Pregnancy

General Precautions: IV access is generally recommended for any injections in the C and T spine, whereas most do not require it for lumbar z-joint blocks (19,20).

Premedication: Premedication is not generally used

Monitoring blood pressure is not considered necessary in lumbar z-joint blocks in a stable patient

Resuscitation equipment should be available

Injection Techniques

All z-joint injection techniques that we describe require several key components. All require knowledge of the spinal anatomy involved. One must then translate the two-dimensional fluoroscopic images seen and develop the art of placing the needle into the three-dimensional spine.

Corticosteroids

There are proponents for Depo-medrol (methylprednisolone acetate), Celestone (betamethasone), and several others. Roughly equivalent dosing would be 40 mg of depomedrol compared to 6 mg of betamethasone. These are injected in very small volumes, e.g., 2–3 mg celestone in 1 ml in lumbar joints and 1–2 mg celestone in 0.4–0.6 ml in cervical joints.

Lumbar Intra-Articular Zygapophyseal Joint Blocks

The patient lies prone under the image intensifier. The target joint must be imaged from the posterior or oblique position. The upper lumbar joints are generally sagittally oriented, whereas the lower segments become more oblique and even more coronal. As a result, the upper lumbar joints can be approached from the posterior approach, whereas the lower levels usually require the patient to roll to a posterior oblique position or tilt the C-arm to bring the joint into view.

A 22-gauge or 25-gauge spinal needle (double needle technique is an option) is guided to the posterior joint using intermittent fluoroscopy. Once the needle touches bone, it is guided into the joint by feel. It is appropriate to guide it deep enough in the joint to ensure entry but not so deep as to limit the ability to inject.

Osteophytes may block entry from the posterior edge of the joint, so alternative approaches include entry through the joint recesses inferiorly or superiorly. Once the joint is entered, a small quantity of dye (0.3 ml) is injected using a 2–5 ml syringe to minimize injection pressure. An arthrogram is noted if the needle is within the joint capsule with flow into the recesses common due to normal capsular foramina (and not rupture). A PA and lateral view is valuable. If dye flows into the multifidus muscle posteriorly, placement must be re-attempted. Once intra-articular injection is achieved, an additional injection of local anesthetic with or without corticosteroid can be added.

Generally, only 1 ml of solution is injected to avoid capsular rupture. If therapeutic benefits are hoped for, intra-articular injections are sought (Figs. 1A–1C).

Lumbar Medial Branch Blocks

For diagnostic purposes, blocking the medial branch at the z joint and the level below is equivalent to blocking the z joint itself. The L1–L4 medial branches of the dorsal ramus have been shown (11) to lie at the junction of the root of the transverse process and root of the superior articular process. Some would call this the "base of the Scotty Dog's Ear" on oblique imaging (Figs. 1D and 1E). The L5 medial branch similarly lies adjacent to the S1 superior articular process at the sacral ala.

A 22- or 25-gauge needle may enter the skin just above the transverse process of the target point. This allows appropriate caudal orientation without being blocked by the mammillary body adjacent to the sulcus. A volume of 0.5 ml should be injected slowly to pool it at the nerve rather than spread out

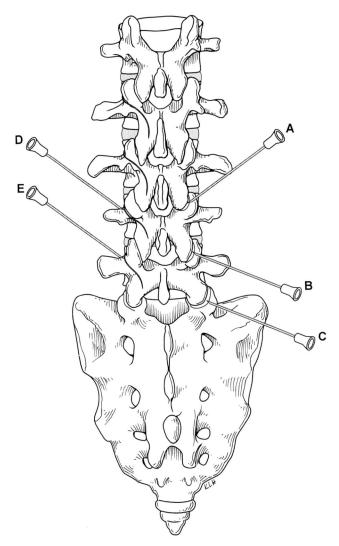

FIG. 1. Lumbar zygapophyseal (facet) joint, and medial branch block needle placement. Lumbar medial branch blocks at D(L4) and E(L5) *(left)*. Both have innervation of the left L4/5 z joint. *(Right):* Z-joint needle placement shown at **A**: right L3/4 z joint. **B**: L4/5 z joint, **C**: L5-S1 z joint. (Reprinted with permission from the State University of New York Health Science Center, Syracuse.)

into muscle or adjacent nerves which would diminish the accuracy of diagnosis.

Complications of Lumbar Spine Blocks

Complications are rare. Usually just local needle or z-joint pain are sequelae. Appropriate care and attention to anatomy under fluoroscopy should minimize the major complications of needle injury to the cord or nerve roots or puncture of the epidural, subdural, or subarachnoid space.

TECHNICAL ASPECTS OF Z-JOINT INJECTIONS: CERVICAL SPINE

Generally, it is recommended that one has extensive experience working in the lumbar spine before progressing on to the C spine.

A posterior approach is recommended for the "typical" intra-articular blocks from C3–4 to C6–7, and possibly C7-T1.

A patient is placed prone on the x-ray table. The face is supported by a doughnut-shaped pillow. It is important that the neck be held in either neutral or a slightly flexed position to ease placement of the needles into the facet joints. The patient should be comfortable with the arms positioned to not interfere with the lateral x-ray images of the involved level. The fluoroscopy unit(s) are then positioned to obtain a true AP and lateral image of the segments to be examined. The neck is then prepared and draped in the standard manner. The z joint should be entered at the cephalic tip of the inferior z-joint and in the lateral half of the z joint itself. This prevents the possibility of entrance into the spinal canal and subsequent epidural or intrathecal injection. With this in mind, the appropriate starting points are first located on the scan using fluoroscopy image.

The needle should start inferior to the joint being injected which eases penetration of the needle into the joint. Attempting to enter the joint from either a straight vertical or from a more cranial position is very difficult and many times can not be accomplished. The usual skin entry point is 1–2 inches (2 or more segments) below the level of the z joint, in line with the z joint itself. Using appropriate biplane technique, the needle is advanced slowly under local anesthesia to the z-joint capsule. Many times a "pop" can be felt as the needle penetrates the capsule and enters the actual joint. An arthrogram confirms location. Local anesthetic with or without steroids can then be injected. The normal joint holds 1/2–1 ml maximum. Recovery following injections is necessary. The patient is observed for the next 30 minutes. If excess or misplaced local anesthetic has leaked into the epidural space, it can produce a high level of block including possible respiratory paralysis.

If the needle were to wander, penetration of the epidural, subdural, or subarachnoid space could occur with its subsequent effects being possible. Minor sequelae may include post-injection pain and light-headedness. Ataxia and dizziness may occur due to the block of proprioceptive and postural input from neck muscles (20) (Figs. 2A and 2B).

The patient's response to the injections, in regard to pain at the time of dye injection, relief of pain from the local anesthetic, and long-term effects, are recorded.

Some have advocated a lateral intra-articular approach with the patient lying on their side. The z joint is identified on a true lateral view and the needle is entered through the skin over the midpoint of the joint. Initially, the needle is directed to touch bone to give the correct depth of injection and then directed through the joint being cautious to avoid overinsertion.

Imaging may be a problem as the lateral view shows both z joints. Rotating the patient or the imaging tube is necessary to identify which side is superior (the side being injected), and must be clarified to prevent cord injury. The lateral approach has the advantage of allowing a shorter course for the needle to travel.

C2–3 intra-articular blocks are best approached using a posterolateral image (8,19). The patient lies on their side and then rotates their head toward the table to open the z-joint cavity to enable direct entry from the posterolateral aspect of the joint.

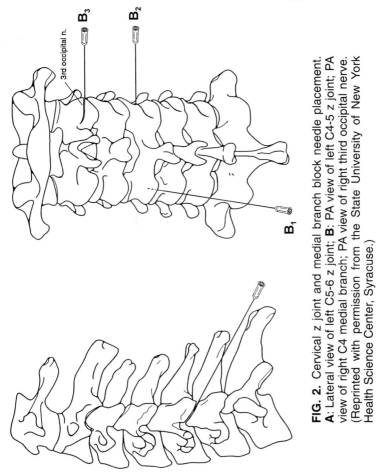

FIG. 2. Cervical z joint and medial branch block needle placement. **A**: Lateral view of left C5-6 z joint; **B**: PA view of left C4-5 z joint; PA view of right C4 medial branch; PA view of right third occipital nerve. (Reprinted with permission from the State University of New York Health Science Center, Syracuse.)

Atlanto-occipital and lateral atlanto axial joint approaches have been described by Bogduk, Dreyfuss, and others for head and neck pain (8,14,18,20). The proximity to the vertebral and internal carotid arteries as well as the dural sac and spinal cord requires great care. The lateral A-A joint is approached posteriorly with the target just lateral to the middle of the joint line. Further research is required to clarify the diagnostic and therapeutic indications for this technique.

CERVICAL MEDIAL BRANCH BLOCKS

When only diagnostic information is being sought, medial branch blocks may be preferable in terms of safety. The needle will be on bone and well away from vital structures. The cervical medial branches C3-C4 through C7-T1 cross the waists of the articular pillars.

POSTERIOR APPROACH

The patient lies prone with a cushion under the head and chest. The PA view shows the z joints as convexities and the concavities are the waists of the articular pillars. A 22-gauge needle is inserted through the skin and muscle to touch the articular pillar just medial to the lateral concavity. Once bone is touched, the needle is walked laterally until it slips ventrally and then brought back to that lateral point which is the site of the segmental medial branch. To block a joint, 0.5 ml of local anesthetic should slowly be injected over 30 to 60 seconds at the medial branch site above and below the z joint.

Lateral Approach

The patient lies on their side and the needle is directed to the mid point of the articular pillar. Once again the lateral projection requires care in determining the uppermost from lower (opposite side) pillar. This can be clarified by slightly rolling the patient or the C-arm (Fig. 3.)

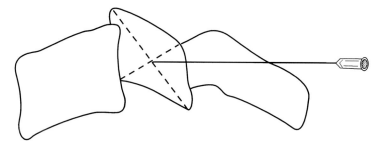

FIG. 3. Landmarks for needle placement in the lateral approach for cervical medial branch blocks (center of trapezoid-shaped lateral body). (Reprinted with permission from the State University of New York Health Science Center, Syracuse.)

Third Occipital Nerve

The third occipital nerve block requires special attention. The C2-3 z joint is innervated by the third occipital nerve which is much thicker than the typical medial branches. This must be blocked at three locations. The posterior approach requires the usual injection at the lateral convexity but also the lowest border of the convexity and another half way between. The lateral approach is best with three injections done in the midline of the C2-3 joint. One at the joint and one just above and the final injection just below the joint line (8,16,20) (Fig. 2, B3).

THORACIC INTRA-ARTICULAR
Z-JOINT BLOCKS

The patient is placed prone with PA imaging. The target z joint cannot be visualized in the PA image. It lies between two consecutive pedicles. It is oriented at a shallow angle with the caudal border at the superior aspect of the lower vertebral pedicle image. The needle is inserted inferior to the joint by starting the skin insertion at the level of the inferior spinous process in line with the pedicle. The needle is slowly advanced to the top of the pedicle feeling for the small dip to the entrance of the facet joint. The needle should not be allowed to wander medially toward the dura and cord or too far laterally to the pleura. When the needle is felt to engage the joint, either a small amount of dye can be injected or the needle can be advanced into the joint until a small bend is noted. A better alternative noted by Dreyfuss is to visualize the lateral joint by rotating the C-arm away from the joint until the lateral joint space is seen with the needle placed (17,20). Once the arthrogram fills, the circular outline of the joint is noted cephalad to the pedicle on PA views. The joint can be injected with local anesthetic with a total of 0.6 ml to prevent rupturing the joint capsule.

Medial branch blocks have been proposed because anatomic studies located the thoracic medial branches by Chua and Bogduk (12b). No studies regarding these blocks have been published to date (Fig. 4).

Sacroiliac Joint Injections

Although this is not a z joint, it is a synovial joint that has potential for back and referred pain. The SI joint is best approached from the lower aspect of the joint. The patient lies prone and the needle is directed to touch the sacrum adjacent to the inferior aspect of the joint line. By touching bone first, the adjacent soft tissues and pelvic contents are avoided and the needle can be directed to the joint. The inferior joint capsule may also be a useful point of entry (Fig. 5). Once the needle is placed in the joint, an auricular shaped arthrogram pattern should be seen. Approximately 2–3 ml total fluid can be instilled, being careful not to rupture the joint capsule. There is also the ligamentous superior aspect of the SI joint that can not be filled and may also be a source for pain.

Aprill, Fortin, and Dreyfuss have presented typical pain patterns (8,14,15,20).

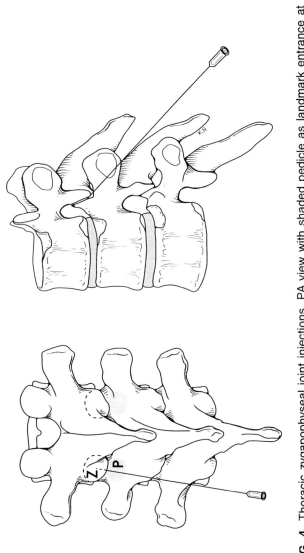

FIG. 4. Thoracic zygapophyseal joint injections. PA view with shaded pedicle as landmark entrance at 11:00–12:00 position at top of pedicle (*P*). Needle placement may be checked by viewing needle from opposite oblique fluoroscopy. Appearance of zygapophyseal (Z) joint (*dotted circle*) on PA not noted until injected with contrast. Lateral view of needle placement illustrating landmarks and flat angle of approach required to enter this joint. (Reprinted with permission from the State University of New York Health Science Center, Syracuse.)

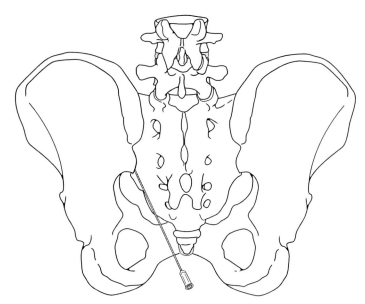

FIG. 5. SI joint needle placement at the inferior medial aspect of the joint. (Reprinted with permission from the State University of New York Health Science Center, Syracuse.)

SUMMARY

Z joints are a potential source for spine pain both locally and referred. Carefully performed z-joint blocks are a definitive method to diagnose this key source of spine pain.

REFERENCES

1. Abel MS. The radiology of chronic neck pain: Sequaelae of occult traumatic lesions. *CRC Crit Rev Diagn Imag* 1982;20:27.
2. Aprill C, Bogduk N. The prevalence of cervical zygapophyseal joint pain: A first approximation. Cervical zygapophyseal joint pain. *Spine* 1992;17:744–747.
3. Aprill C, Dwyer A, Bogduk N. Cervical zygapophyseal joint pain patterns II: A clinical evaluation. *Spine* 1990;15:458–461.
4. Barnsley L, Lord S, Bogduk N. Clinical review—Whiplash injury. *Pain* 1994;58:283–307.
5. Barnsley L, Lord S, Bogduk N. Comparative local anaesthetic blocks in the diagnosis of cervical zygapophyseal joint pain. *Pain* 1993;55:99–106.

6. Barnsley L, Lord S, Wallis B, Bogduk N. Lack of effect of intraarticular corticosteroids for chronic pain in the cervical zygapophyseal joints. Intra-articular corticosteroid injections after whiplash. *N Engl J Med* 1994;330:1047–1050.

7. Barnsley L, Lord S, Wallis B, Bogduk N. The prevalence of chronic cervical zygapophyseal joint pain after whiplash. *Spine* 1995;20:20–26.

8. Bogduk N, Aprill C, Derby R. Diagnostic blocks of spinal synovial joints. In: White A, ed. *Spine Care*. Mosby, St. Louis; 1995.

9. Bogduk N, Long D. Percutaneous lumbar medial branch neurotomy: A modification of facet denervation. *Spine* 1980;5:193–200.

10. Bogduk N. *Spine Supplement* [Editorial]. 1995;20:8S–9S.

11. Bogduk N. The innervation of the lumbar spine. *Spine* 1983;8:286–293.

12a. Carette S, Marcoux S, Truchon R, et al. A controlled trial of corticosteroid injections into facet joints for chronic low back pain. *N Engl J Med* 1991;325:1002.

12b. Chua W, Bogduk N. *The surgical anatomy of the thoracic dorsal rami*. Presented at the ISIS 2nd Annual Meeting, Minneapolis, Minnesota; 1994.

13. Derby R, Kine G, Schofferman, Bogduk N, Ronnow S. *A prospective evaluation of medial branch neurotomy for zygapophyseal joint (z joint pain)*. Presented at the Annual Meeting of the North American Spine Society, Washington D.C.; 1995.

14. Derby R, Bogduk N, Schwarzer A. Precision percutaneous blocking procedures for localizing spinal pain. Part 1: The posterior lumbar compartment. *Pain Digest* 1993;3:89–100.

15. Derby R, Kine G, Aprill C. *International Spine Injection Society Workshop for Lumbar Spine Injection Techniques*. Daly City, Calif.; 1994.

16. Derby R, Kine G, Aprill C. *International Spine Injection Society Workshop for Cervical/Thoracic Injection Treatments*. Daly City, Calif., 1995.

17. Dreyfuss P, Tibiletti C, Dreyer S. Thoracic zygapophyseal joint pain patterns: A study in normal volunteers. *Spine* 1994;19:807–811.

18. Dreyfuss P, Michaelsen M, Fletcher D. Atlanto-occipital and lateral atlanto-axial joint pain patterns. *Spine* 1994;19:1125–1131.

19. Dreyfuss P, Dreyer S, Herring S. Contemporary concepts in spine care lumbar zygapophyseal (facet) joint injections. *Spine* 1995;20:2040–2047.

20. Dreyfuss P, Lagattuta F, Kaplansky B, Heller B. Zygapophyseal joint injection techniques in the spinal axis. In: *Physiatric procedures in clinical practice*. Mosby, St. Louis; 1995.

21. Dwyer A, Aprill C, Bogduk N. Cervical zygapophyseal joint pain patterns I: Study in normal volunteers. *Spine* 1990;15:453–457.

22. Esses S, Moro J. The value of facet joint blocks in patient selection for lumbar fusion. *Spine* 1993;18:183–190.

23. Fairbank JCT, Park WM, McCall IW, O'Brien JP. Apophyseal injection of local anesthetic as a diagnostic aid in primary low-back pain syndromes. *Spine* 1981;6:598.

24a. Helbig T, Lee CK. The lumbar facet syndrome. *Spine* 13:61, 198.

24b. Jackson R. The facet syndrome-myth or reality? *Clinical Orthopaedics and Related Research* 1992;279:110–121.

25. Klein R, Eek B, Delong B, Mooney V. A randomized double blind trial of dextrose, glycerine and phenol injections for chronic low back pain. *J Spine Dis* 1993;6:23–33.
26. Lilius G, Laasonen EM, Myllynen P, et al. Lumbar facet joint syndrome: A randomised clinical trial. *J Bone Joint Surg* 1989;71B:681.
27. Lippit AB. The facet joint and its role in spine pain: Management with facet joint injections. *Spine* 1984;9:746.
28. Little F. Renewed considerations in the diagnosis and treatment of degenerative zygapophyseal (facet) joint, primary discogenic, and intrinsic nerve root pain syndromes of the lower back and extremities. *Neurosurgery Quarterly* 1993;3:1–39.
29. Lord S, Barnsley L, Bogduk N. Cervical zygapophyseal joint pain in whiplash. *Spine: State of the Art Reviews* 1993;7:355–372.
30. Mooney V, Robertson J. The facet syndrome. *Clin Ortho* 1976;115:149.
31. Schwarzer A, Aprill C, Derby R, Fortin J, Kine G, et al. Clinical features of patients with pain stemming from the lumbar zygapophyseal joints: Is the lumbar facet syndrome a clinical entity? *Spine* 1994;19:1132–1137.
32. Schwarzer AC, Aprill CN, Derby K, Fortin J, Kine G, Bogduk N. The false positive rate of uncontrolled diagnostic blocks of the lumbar zygapophyseal joints. *Pain* 1994;58:195–200.
33. Schwarzer A, Wang S, O'Driscoll D, Harrington T, Bodguk N, et al. The ability of computed tomography to identify a painful zygapophyseal joint in patients with chronic low back pain. *Spine* 1995;20:907–912.
34. Schwarzer A, Aprill C, Derby R, Fortin J, Kine G, et al. The relative contributions of the disc zygapophyseal joint and chronic low back pain. *Spine* 1994;19:801–806.
35. Stolker, Vervest A, Groen G. The management of chronic spine pain block by blockades: A review. *Pain* 1994;58:1–20.
36. Ottolengi C. Aspiration biopsy of the spine. *J Bone Joint Surg* 1969; 51A:1531–1544.

IMAGE-GUIDED PAIN MANAGEMENT
edited by P. S. Thomas.
Lippincott–Raven Publishers, Philadelphia © 1997

19

Discography

Thomas D. Masten and Bruce E. Fredrickson

*Department of Orthopedic Surgery, SUNY Health Science Center at
Syracuse, Syracuse, New York 13210*

TERMINOLOGY

Discography is the injection of radiographic dye into the nucleus of an intervertebral disc, which is then imaged. Disc puncture, injection of the dye, documenting the response of the patient to the injection (i.e., recording pain provocation), imaging with plain radiograph and/or CT are all considered integral parts of discography.

HISTORY

Discography was first described in the 1940s (22,29) as a method to image the disc. The only alternative of confirming a disc herniation at that time was imaging the outer aspect of the disc covered by dura by doing myelography. With the advent of computerized tomography (CT) and later magnetic resonance imaging (MRI), diagnostic imaging has been markedly improved. However, discography has maintained its value because it has the unique ability to determine if a disc is the actual source of pain.

Discography has been very controversial since it was first described. Although there has been excellent evidence to support its use (2,6,19), it still remains a source of controversy. Key reasons for the controversy have been issues of safety and

151

validity. The current improved techniques, imaging, and contrast dyes have been shown to be safe (6,16,19). Earlier studies which raised concerns regarding validity (23) have been countered with newer studies that are reassuring (43,46).

LOCATING THE SOURCE OF SPINE PAIN

Anatomy

All three compartments of the spine (posterior, neuraxial, and anterior) are believed to be potential sources for pain. The anterior compartment includes the vertebra and the discs (6). The cervical and lumbar discs receive innervation to the annulus. The posterior innervation of the disc is from the sinovertebral nerves, laterally from the vertebral nerve and anteriorly from the sympathetic nerves. The thoracic disc is probably similar but anatomists are still defining that more clearly. The main purpose of disc injection is to determine which disc is the symptomatic source of pain in a particular patient.

Imaging

With the steady improvement of CT and MRI, imaging of the pathology has improved. With the description of the high intensity zone (HIZ), best seen on T2-weighted image, annular fissures could be found (3). In 1989, Yu (50) found lumbar discography more sensitive than MRI for detection of annular fissures. In 1994, however, Ito and Yu (24) found MRI was a bit more sensitive than discography for finding radial tears, but it was not very specific for which would be painful. In fact, loss of disc height and severe disc degeneration were found to be better predictors of painful disc levels.

EVALUATION OF PERSISTENT SPINAL PAIN

Discography is an uncomfortable, often painful invasive diagnostic intervention. It should not be used until conservative therapy has failed to adequately address the patient's symptoms. If MRI or CT fail to yield sufficient information, discography has several valuable contributions.

Discography may be helpful in patients who have clinical findings suggestive of disc pathology, but is insufficient diagnostic information. There are instances when a patient may have severe spinal pain possibly with referred or radicular symptoms with minimal or no disc bulge on imaging. A discogram may outline an annular tear, with typical pain provocation even into a limb in the disc disruption syndrome.

Another instance is when there is a need to correlate imaging with clinical symptoms. Disc bulges at multiple levels may require a discogram to clarify if one or more levels generate the spinal pain of concern to the patient. Lateral disc herniations (e.g., foraminal or extraforaminal) may be a source of spinal pain best evaluated by discography (25,28).

An interesting new concept has been the use of a careful McKenzie mechanical (physical therapy) assessment to forecast the outcomes of discography (4). This assessment may act as a "functional" discogram and offer a less invasive alternative to obtain some of the information thought only available by discography prior to this study.

Improving Surgical Outcomes

Prior to surgery, especially a fusion, assessment of the spine by discography may prove helpful. The principal source(s) of pain may be found as well as evaluating adjacent discs to study their integrity by noting the degree of degeneration.

With minimally invasive surgical interventions, discography has been of value to clarify if a disc is contained. Sequestered discs may not be managed well by some techniques.

Prior Fusion Surgery With Persistent Symptoms

Sorting out the source of pain following fusion may be possible with discography even in patients with a solid posterior fusion (48). Painful pseudarthrosis post fusion may be evaluated with discography to determine if the problem is with the level that failed to fuse or an adjacent level (26b).

Special Clinical Concerns

Recurrent disc herniation may be best demonstrated by discogram. Guyer found CT discogram showed disc herniations not visualized with gadolinium enhanced MRI (19).

Kostuik has found discography valuable in choosing between anterior or posterior fusion in adult scoliosis with improved pain relief (27b).

Medicolegal

Some feel that the discogram can be used to objectively establish the source of pain in medicolegal cases.

Contraindications

Bleeding diatheses
Infection
Drug Allergy

Precautions/Complications

The main complications of discography are discitis (disc infection) and neural injury. Other complications have included spinal cord or nerve root injury, urticaria, retroperitoneal hemorrhage, nausea, convulsions, headache, and most commonly, increased pain (19).

Based on a study by Fraser (15), some prefer using a double needle technique. However, note that the single needle approach described in that study used an open needle with no stylet (2). Others still prefer a single needle technique using a needle with a stylet.

Discitis is usually considered with the onset of severe axial spine pain days to weeks following disc puncture.

Some prefer to use antibiotics in the performance of discography based on a study by Osti (35). Cervical discography has the additional rare risks for epidural abscess, retropharyngeal abscess (2), injection-induced disc herniation, and subdural empyema (19). In the cervical region, oropharyngeal bacteria are often implicated (8).

Pneumothorax is a potential risk for discography at C7 down through the thorax. Cord compression or myelopathy adds too great a risk for discography due to potential severe consequences (2). The complication of cervical cord puncture has been reported by some with variable outcomes. Patients have described severe pain but no neurologic sequelae with discography (2), as well as with cervical puncture for myelography (34).

Disc Damage

Grubb reported one instance of disc herniation following discography in a series of 346 disc injections (18).

Techniques

Lumbar Disc Puncture (2,6)

Patient preparation includes a screening history, exam, and informed consent (including an explanation of the procedure, risks, and benefits), and premedication if indicated.

Our approach utilizes biplane fluoroscopy, although C-arm is similarly useful allowing true PA and lateral views. Some advocate a single PA tower, with movement of the patient to obtain PA, lateral, or oblique views. Although this is possible, it is also more time consuming, and moving the patient may change the needle position.

The patient is initially placed in the prone position and is thoroughly prepped from the ribs to the mid-sacral level from the spine to the mid-axillary line on the side opposite to the patient's major distal pain. If the pain is radiating down the left leg, then the injection is approached from the right side. This is done to minimize confusing the patient's typical pain location with the pain which might be produced by needle placement adjacent to the neural elements or leakage of dye through the needle tract.

Exceptions to this positioning may occur due to anatomic variations such as dilated dural nerve root sleeve or composite nerve root sleeve on the side you wish to approach (2). In these cases, injection may best be carried out on the painful side.

In the past, a midline (posterior/between the pedicles) approach has been used by some, but this approach assumes the risks of dural puncture and is not preferred in our institution. The lateral approach external to the pedicle is used with a much lower risk of dural puncture, however, neural injury by direct trauma may occur. A report of bowel puncture has occurred when using an extreme lateral approach (5).

There are several variations available for the extrapedicular approach. The prone approach is also useful when using larger instruments for percutaneous procedures. The prone oblique technique will be described as well. Some prefer a lateral approach which may be helpful in maneuvering around posterior fusions but will not be described.

The prone lateral approach may be easier if the lateral image is used to aid in marking the disc levels on the patient's skin prior to prepping. A starting point about 6 to 8 cm from the midline at the level of the disc is then numbed with local anesthetic. When using a double needle technique, an 18- or 20-gauge 3- to 6-inch needle with a stylet is then directed to the disc. The true PA image of parallel endplates is then used to gauge the needle direction toward the inferior half of the disc (to avoid the exiting nerve root). With this position in mind, the depth of the needle is determined on the lateral image. By "triangulating" from these two images the needle can be slowly guided to the disc making directional adjustments as needed. The needle course can be guided by moving the point of the needle (opposite to the bevel) toward the target point. If a bony endpoint is felt, the imaging must determine if this a posterior element or the vertebral endplate adjacent to the disc.

Usually a small rotation of the needle can alter the direction, whereas at other times, a carefully planned partial withdrawal of the needle with redirection is needed.

Once the posterior elements are passed or the annulus is contacted with a firm but resilient endpoint, the stylet is removed. The smaller gauge, longer needle (e.g., a 22-gauge 6-inch needle is placed within the 3-inch 18-gauge "sleeve" needle, although some prefer a 25-gauge needle inside a 20-gauge sleeve). Some find the movement of the procedure needle is more easily directed if it has been slightly angled by hand using a sterile gauze to maintain sterility of the tip. This allows more control of movement of the needle tip in guiding it to the middle third of the disc to reach the nucleus (Fig. 1).

This approach works well for the lumbar discs above L5-S1. The lumbosacral junction requires a starting point adjacent to the L4–L5 insertion point to avoid the iliac crest. The needle can then be directed to the disc at an oblique angle.

Posterior Oblique Approach

The initial preparation is the same in this approach. The posterior oblique approach differs in that the patient is placed in the lateral decubitus position with the painful side down and the side to be approached up. Various padding and pillows can help the patient to be comfortable in this position including a pillow under the head, a bolster to diminish side bending and the hip and knee (on the side to be injected) can be flexed. The patient is rolled until the optimal fluoroscopic view is obtained. In this technique, the key is to locate the superior articular process of the lower vertebra.

Rotate the patient so the superior articular process is placed 1/3 to 1/2 of the way between the margins of the vertebra, in the true PA view. A 22- to 25-gauge 3 1/2-inch spinal needle can be advanced to the anterior base of the superior articular

A.

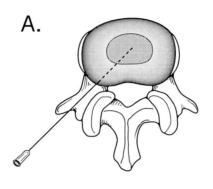

B.

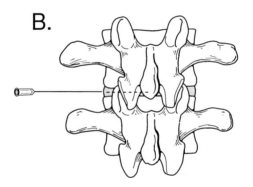

C.

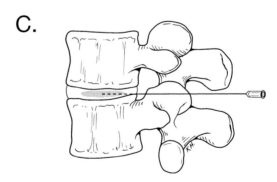

FIG. 1. Importance of biplane *(PA and Lateral)* fluoroscopy guided views in needle placement in lumbar discography; **A–C,** shows perfect placement of needle in disc nucleus on A *(cross section)*, B *(true PA)*, C *(true lateral)*.

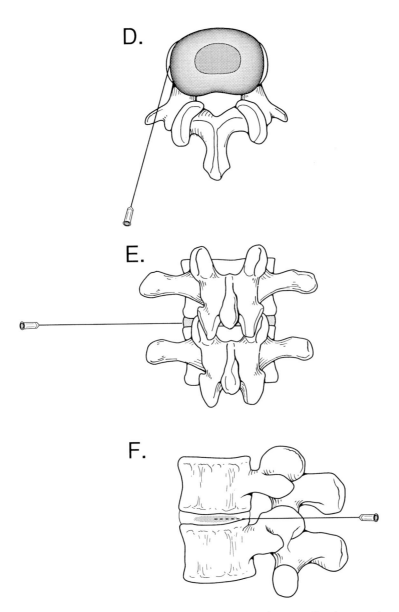

FIG. 1. D–F, shows that what appears to be perfect needle placement on the lateral view (D) is, in fact, far lateral on the PA view and on cross-sectional illustration.

process to establish direction, depth, and to numb the needle tract to the bone through fascia. The same double needle technique noted can then be used to achieve disc puncture. One author finds it easier to negotiate past the posterior elements using this technique (Fig. 2).

Once again, the L5-S1 disc presents a special challenge requiring a modification in technique (2). This time the patient is rotated to a prone or near prone position to allow the image of the lateral aspect of the superior process to be seen just medial to the iliac crest. A 22- to 25-gauge needle can be guided to the superior edge of the sacrum so the depth and direction can be determined and the soft tissues can be anes-

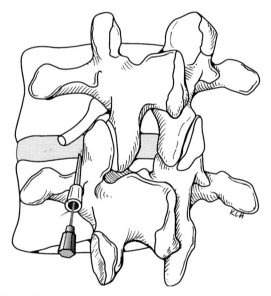

FIG. 2. Illustration of the oblique approach to lower lumbar discography. The patient is in the left posterior oblique position. The leading edge of the superior articular processes positioned 1/3 to 1/2 the distance between the borders of the vertebral body as viewed on fluoroscopy. The sleeve needle with stylet is guided to the junction of the superior articular process and transverse process, and then guided just superior to the endplate into the "safe triangle." The stylet is removed and the procedure needle punctures the disc and is advanced into the nucleus. (Reprinted with permission from SUNY Health Science Center, Syracuse, New York.)

thetized with local anesthetic. The angle should be in line with the disc space on lateral imaging. Next, the large gauge (e.g., 18 gauge) spinal needle which is to act as the sleeve needle is advanced to this position at the anterolateral edge of the superior articular process of the sacrum. The needle is then walked off the bone but stopped at that point.

A precurved procedure needle (e.g., a 6-inch 22-gauge needle), is placed within the larger gauge spinal needle after removing the 18-gauge needle stylet. The curve must be more pronounced at this level than at the more superior levels. Care must be taken as the L5 nerve root lies in close proximity. The lateral view allows clarification of depth. If the procedure needle is too far anterior, it may require withdrawing the procedure needle inside the sleeve needle and backing out the sleeve needle slightly to allow more of a curve to develop in the procedure needle. Once disc puncture is achieved, the needle tip is carefully guided to the central third of the disc to reach the nucleus. This technique often allows a more easy entry to the lumbosacral disc even in an individual with a high pelvic brim or in more obese individuals (although a 6-inch sleeve needle and 8-inch procedure needle may be required).

Pain Response

The pain response to the disc injection is extremely important. The pain severity and location at the time of injection separates discography from all other imaging available for the disc. Although pain severity and the response to pain may have emotional and subjective overlay, a patient can usually compare his/her own degree of pain prior to injection with that noted post injection. The location or change in location of the pain in response to injection seems objective as well.

The objective observation of pain response is our goal. The chronic pain being studied is compared to the pain produced by the injection of solution into the nucleus. Various responses are possible. VanHaranta, et al. (46) described one method of classifying the pain. There may be (a) no pain, or pressure only, (b) pain dissimilar to clinical symptoms, (c) pain similar to clini-

cal symptoms, (d) exact reproduction of symptoms. Pain intensity may be recorded on an analog or 0–10 scale comparing
pre- and post-injection pain. Nonspecific pain behavior is felt
to be of significance with objectivity by some observers (47)
who also note grimacing, rubbing, verbalizing, guarding, withdrawal, and sighing.

The comparison of a painful disc to an adjacent disc which
is normal is felt to be important. In this way, a patient's
response to injection in a normal disc can be used as baseline
or control for injections at other disc levels.

Discography

Once the needle tip is in the center of the disc, a 1 to 5 ml
syringe is used to inject contrast. The volume accepted and the
quality of the resistance is noted. A normal disc will accept 1.5
to 2.5 ml of fluid with a cottonball appearance.

The appearance of the dye when injected in the nucleus
(nucleogram) is valuable information. Various terms have been
used to describe the appearance of the nucleus (1,24,39,50,51).
Normal discs have a globular "cottonball" appearance or a
bilobed "hamburger" appearance. If the nuclear appearance is
irregular flowing into fissures, tears may be described as radial,
circumferential, or transverse. The dye may be contained
within the disc, extend to the outermost annulus, or leak out of
the annulus into the epidural space or through the cartilaginous
endplate into the vertebral body. A single thin tear to the posterolateral outermost annulus may produce lateralizing pain.
Ito (24) has shown that generally degenerated discs are most
likely to be pain sources (Fig. 3).

Pain Relief, Analgesic Discography

Analgesic discography has been used as an adjunct to pain
response. After pain provocation during the injection of solution into the nucleus, imaging is carried out with dye in the
disc. If typical pain is produced during the injection and it is

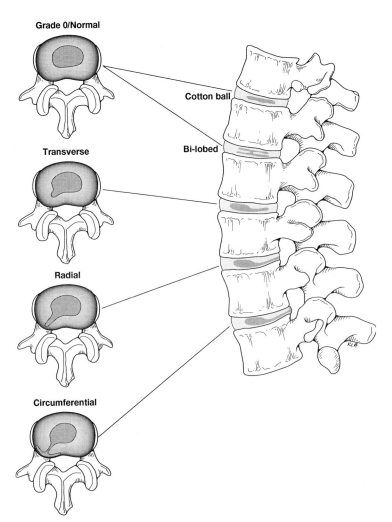

FIG. 3. Illustration of patterns of internal disc disruption Grade 0/Normal—may be either "Cottonball" or Bilobed appearance. Transverse tears appear to extend to the inner fibers of the annulus. Radial tears extend to the outer annulus. Circumferential tears extend between layers of the annulus. (Reprinted with permission from SUNY Health Science Center, Syracuse, New York.)

then resolved by injection of local anesthetic, some feel this is added evidence to support that particular disc is the source for pain. This is more often a clear finding in cervical analgesic discography (38). Others (2) have also attempted injection of therapeutic substances to obtain relief from intradiscal pain. Corticosteroids have been supported by some (49), both for diminishing the discomfort of the test as well as giving longer relief to a subset of patients.

Cervical Disc Puncture (2,6)

Pre-procedural evaluation and explanation of the procedure is again important for this uncomfortable, and at times, very painful procedure. Special caution to remain NPO is noted due to the proximity of the esophagus. An anterior approach is used. The patient lies supine on the fluoroscopy table. Neck extension is required for the procedure but neutral posture may be maintained until the procedure begins to avoid pain exacerbation. True PA and lateral imaging is required, using either a biplane fluoroscopy unit, C-arm, or a combination of a fixed PA unit and a lateral C-arm. Biplane fluoroscopy allows a quicker and more efficient procedure if it is available.

Aseptic technique is once again required with sterile prep and draping of the anterior neck from the mandible to the clavicle. Draping the shoulders is useful to allow the operator to help in depressing the shoulders in viewing the lower C-spine.

It is important to be sure the disc level to be studied can be visualized in PA and lateral views before attempting puncture. No sedation is used in our institution but premedication is used by some (e.g., midazolam). The patient must be able to respond to directions and questions regarding the pain location and distribution.

The neck is usually approached from the right to take advantage of the anatomic positioning of the esophagus to the left in the lower neck. Full neck extension is achieved with a pillow or bolster under the shoulders with the chin raised. The level to be studied is identified under fluoroscopy. The index and middle finger are gently but firmly placed to move the laryngotracheal and esophageal structures medially and the carotid artery (internal above C4 and common below C4) laterally. The anterior spine can usually be palpated. The medial border of the sternocleidomastoid guides the location of the puncture to avoid the pharynx superiorly (above C3-4) and the apex of the lung inferiorly. If needles larger than 25-gauge will be used, it may be best to use local anesthetic on the skin. Using either a spinal needle with stylet or a double needle technique, a small gauge (20-gauge sleeve, with 25-gauge procedure needle placed inside or single 3 1/2-inch 22- or 25-gauge needle) is placed. The procedure needle is advanced obliquely to the anterior spine. The initial target is the superior aspect of the vertebra just below the disc to be studied. When contact with bone is safely made to determine its depth, the needle can be slightly withdrawn and redirected or "walked" into the anterior disc annulus. Although both the periosteum and annulus are innervated and uncomfortable to touch, no local is used to avoid altering the pain response to the disc injection. The needle is carefully advanced into the disc under direct visualization as to avoid passing through the disc (2) (Figs. 4 and 5).

Once the needle tip has been guided to the center of the disc, the dye solution is slowly injected until it enters the nucleus. Visible separation of the vertebra may occur with small volumes (0.2–0.5 ml). Pain response is recorded during this distension. The volume accepted and the quality of the resistance is noted. A normal disc has a firm resistance with less than 0.5 ml and minimal discomfort.

Analgesic discography was introduced as another way to clarify pain response to disc injection (38). Others (49) inject corticosteroids in hopes of long term benefit.

Nucleograms

There is a significant difference between the expected findings in lumbar discograms and those found in the cervical spine. Although a normal nucleus may have only a central lobular nucleus, the findings of posterolateral clefts are normally found over the age of 20. The uncovertebral joints (also named

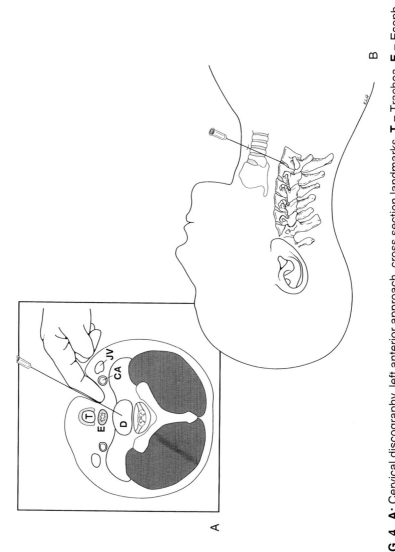

FIG. 4. A: Cervical discography, left anterior approach, cross section landmarks. **T** = Trachea, **E** = Esophagus, **CA** = Carotid Artery, **JV** = Jugular Vein, and **D** = Cervical Disc. **B:** Lateral view of needle placed in C6–7 disc. (Reprinted with permission from SUNY Health Science Center, Syracuse, New York.)

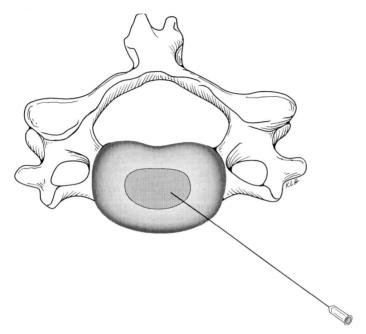

FIG. 5. Cross-section close-up of placement in nucleus.

for Luschka) or articulations, are the attenuated disc annulus that can be fissures in the annulus that communicate with the nucleus. This is a normal maturation process in the cervical disc. As a result, these findings on a nucleogram becomes less important but pain provocation is, therefore, even more note-worthy.

THORACIC DISC PUNCTURE

Technique for Thoracic Discography Using CT Guidance

Although CT-guided techniques can be used in other areas, currently, we only recommend it for the thoracic spine discography. Although it requires CT technology, it improves the safety of the procedure.

The patient is placed on the CT scanner in the prone position. Care is taken to insure comfort of the patient so that they do not require movement during the procedure itself. Using the AP and lateral scout the appropriate disc is determined, and with the axial image the appropriate pathway can be ascertained. Changing the angle of the gantry is at times useful during the axial cuts to insure a parallel entry into the disc space. The laser light is then used to mark the skin at the appropriate level of entry and the appropriate angle of entry can be determined from the axial cuts. The distance from the mid-line that the needle should start can likewise be measured directly off the axial cuts and the distance required before the disc is encountered can likewise be ascertained. The needle is then placed, using a double needle technique. After entering through the skin the needle is advanced approximately 1 to 1 1/2 inches. Using the scout capability, AP and lateral scouts are obtained ensuring proper placement of the needle. The scout x-rays are used in place of the axial x-ray as the needle may not be exactly parallel with the axial image. Therefore, the true degree of penetration of the needle may not be ascertained from the axial cuts during this portion of the procedure. The needle is advanced in gradual increments of 1/2 to 1 inch until it is just outside the disc space. Axial cuts are then taken across the disc space. These cuts are 3 to 5 mm thick and should cover several centimeters to ensure that the true depth of the needle penetration can be ascertained. The inner smaller gauged needle is then used to penetrate the actual disc and placed in the center of the disc. Contrast material is then injected. Pain response of the patient is noted along with the morphologic anatomy of the disc (Fig. 6).

Appropriate scout films and CT cuts are then accomplished. The needles are withdrawn and the patient is observed for the next 1/2 hour before they are allowed to ambulate and be discharged.

A technique described by Schellas (40) uses only fluoroscopy. The target point is the space superior and adjacent to the rib articulation as the patient is brought to the oblique position. A group of 100 patients with clinically suspect abnormal

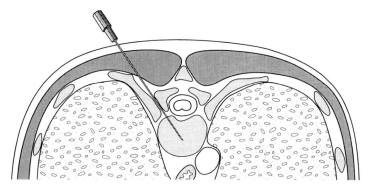

FIG. 6. Cross-section thoracic discography. Needle placement posterior to rib. (Reprinted with permission from SUNY Health Science Center, Syracuse, New York.)

discs on MRI were studied to clarify the source for pain. This was found to be a safe and reliable technique for confirming thoracic disc sources for pain.

Post Procedure Care (2)

Immediate post procedure, the patient is observed for any problems. Most patients can be studied on an outpatient basis and can be discharged after observation. If sedation is used, they must be sufficiently recovered. Patients must have a driver who can observe them and report any problems. Post procedure local pain is usually most noted for 24 to 48 hours and eases over the next 1 to 7 days. Ice packs to minimize bruising may be helpful. Discomfort with swallowing is often noted in those with cervical discography. Asking the patient to keep a pain diary over 7 to 14 days may be helpful to monitor the patients status. A progressive increase or sudden change in the severity of pain should stimulate re-evaluation.

REFERENCES

1. Adams MA, Dolan P, Hutton WC. The stages of disc degeneration as revealed by discograms. *J Bone Joint Surg (Br)* 1986;68:36–41.

2. Aprill C. Diagnostic disc injection. In: Frymoyer J., ed. *The adult spine: Principles and practice.* Raven Press, New York 1991:403–443.
3. Aprill C, Bogduk N. High-intensity zone: A diagnostic sign of painful lumbar disc of magnetic resonance imaging. *Brit J Radiol* 1992;65:361–369.
4. Aprill C, Medcalf R, Donelson R, Grant W, Incorvaia K. *Discographic outcomes predicted by pain centralization and "directional preference": A prospective, blinded study.* Presented at the Annual Meeting of the North American Spine Society, Washington, D.C.; 1995.
5. Benoist M. Positioning alternatives for chemonucleolysis: Current concepts in chemonucleolysis. *J R Soc Med* 1984;72:47–53.
6. Bogduk N, Aprill C, Derby R. Discography. In: White A., ed. *Spine care.* 1995;1:219–238.
7. Brightbill TC, Pile N, Eichelberger R, Whitman M. Normal magnetic resonance imaging and abnormal discography in lumbar disc disruption. *Spine* 1994;19:1075–1077.
8. Cloward R. Cervical diskography—A contribution to the etiology and mechanism of neck, shoulder and arm pain. *Annal Surg* 1959;150:1052–1064.
9. Colhoun E, McCall IW, Williams L, Pullicino VNC. Provocation discography as a guide to planning operations on the spine. *J Bone Joint Surg (Br)* 1988;70:267–271.
10. Collins HR. An evaluation of cervical and lumbar discography. *Clin Orthop* 1975;107:133–138.
11. Connor P, Darden II B. Cervical discography complications and clinical efficacy. *Spine* 1993;18:2035–2038.
12. Derby R, Bogduk N, Kine G. Precision percutaneous blocking procedures for localizing spinal pain, Part 2: The lumbar neuroaxial compartment. *Pain Dig* 1993;3:175–188.
13. Fischgrund J, Montgomery D. Diagnosis and treatment of discogenic low back pain. *Orthopedic Rev* 1993; March:311–318.
14. Flanagan MN, Chung BU. Roentgenographic changes in 188 patients 10–20 years after discography and chemonucleolysis. *Spine* 1986;11:444–448.
15. Fraser RD, Osti OL, Vernon-Roberts B. Discitis after discography. *J Bone Joint Surg (Br)* 1987;69:31–35.
16. Fraser RD, Osti OL, Vernon-Roberts B. Iatrogenic discitis: The role of intravenous antibiotics in prevention and treatment: An experimental study. *Spine* 1989;14:1025.
17. Gill K, Jackson R. CT discography-complications. In: Frymoyer J, ed. *The adult spine: Principles and practice.* Raven Press, New York 1991:444–454.
18. Grubb SA, Lipscomb HJ, Guilford WB. The relative value of lumbar roentgenograms, metrizamide myelography, and discography in the assessment of patients with chronic low back syndrome. *Spine* 1987;12:282–286.
19. Guyer R, Ohnmeiss D. Contemporary concepts in spine care lumbar discography. *Spine* 1995;20:2048–2059.
20. Guyer RD, Collier R, Stith WJ, et al. Discitis after discography. *Spine* 1988;13:1352–1354.

21. Hirsch C. An attempt to diagnose the level of a disc lesion clinically by disc puncture. *Acta Orthop Scand* 1948;18:132–140.
22. Hirsch C. An attempt to diagnose the level of a disc lesion clinically by disc puncture. *Acta Orthop Scand* 1949;18:132.
23. Holt EP. The question of lumbar diskography. *J Bone Joint Surg* [Abstract]. 1968;50:720.
24. Ito M, Incorvaia K, Yu S, Fredrickson B, Yuan H, Rosenbaum R. *Predictive signs of discogenic lumbar pain on MRI with discography correlation.* Presented at the International Society for the Study of the Lumbar Spine, Seattle, Washington; 1994.
25. Jackson RP, Glah JJ. Foraminal and extraforaminal lumbar disc herniation: Diagnosis and treatment. *Spine* 1987;12:577–585.
26a.Johnson RG. Does discography injure normal discs? An analysis of repeat discograms. *Spine* 1989;14:424–426.
26b.Johnson RG, Macnab I. Localization of symptomatic lumbar pseudo arthrosis by use of discography. *Clin Orthop* 1985;197:164–170.
27a.Jonnson H, Bring G, Rauschning W, Sahlstedt B. Hidden cervical spine injuries in traffic accident victims with skull fractures. *J Spinal Disorders* 1991;4:251.
27b.Kostuik JP. Decision making in adult scoliosis. *Spine* 1979;4:521–525.
28. Kurobane Y, Takahashi T, Tajima T, et al. Extraforaminal disc herniation. *Spine* 1986;11:260–268.
29. Lindblom K. Diagnostic puncture of intervertebral disks in sciatica. *Acta Orthop Scand* 1948;17:213–239.
30. Lindblom K. Discography of dissecting transosseous ruptures of intervertebral discs in the lumbar region. *Acta Radiol* 1951;38:96.
31. Mason S, Shelokov A, Guyer R, Ohnmeiss D. *Complications of cervical discography: Findings in a large series.* Presented at the Annual Meeting of the North American Spine Society, Washington D.C.; 1995.
32. McCulloch JA, Waddell G. Lateral lumbar discography. *Br J Radiol* 1978;51:498–502.
33. Moneta GB, Videman T, Kaivento K, Aprill C, Spivey M, et al. Reported pain during lumbar discography as a function of anular ruptures and disk degeneration: A re-analysis of 833 discograms. *Spine* 1994;19:1968–1974.
34. Nakstad PH, Kjartansson O. Accidental spinal cord injection of contrast material during cervical myelograph with C1-Cs puncture. *Am J Neuroradiology* 1988;13:1343.
35. Otsi OL, Fraser RD, Vernon-Roberts B. Discitis after discography: The role of prophylactic antibiotics. *J Bone Joint Surg (Br)* 1990;72:271–274.
36. Parfenchuck T, Janssen M. A correlation of cervical magnetic resonance imaging and discography/computed tomographic discograms. *Spine* 1994;19:2819–2825.
37. Rhyne III A, Smith S, Wood K, Darden II B. Outcome of unoperated discogram-positive low back pain. *Spine* 1995;20:1997–2001.
38. Roth DA. Cervical analgesic discography: A new test for the definitive diagnosis of the painful disc syndrome. *JAMA* 1976;235:1713.
39. Sachs B, Vanharanta H, Spivey M, et al. Dallas discogram description a new classification of CT/discography in low-back disorders. *Spine* 1987;12:287–294.

40. Schellhas K, Pollei S, Dorwart R. Thoracic discography—A safe and reliable technique. *Spine* 1994;19:2103–2109.
41. Schellhas K, Smith M, Gundry C, Pollei S. *Cervical discogenic pain: Prospective correlation of MR imaging and discography.* Presented at the Annual Meeting of the North American Spine Society, Washington D.C.; 1995.
42. Schwarzer A, Aprill C, Derby R, Fortin J, Kine G, et al. The prevalence and clinical features of internal disc disruption in patients with chronic low back pain. *Spine* 1995;20:1878–1883.
43. Simmons J, Aprill C, Dwyer A, Brodsky A. A reassessment of Holt's data on "the question of lumbar discography." *Clin Orthopaed Related Res* 1988;237:120–124.
44. VanHaranta H, Guyer RD, Ohnmeiss DD. Disc deterioration in low-back syndromes: A prospective, multi-center CT/discography study. *Spine* 1988;13:1349–1351.
45. VanHaranta H, Sachs BL, Ohnmeiss DD. Pain provocation and disc deterioration by age. A CT/discography study in a low back pain population. *Spine* 1989;14:420–424.
46. VanHaranta H, Sachs BL, Spivey MA, et al. The relationship of pain provocation to lumbar disc deterioration as seen by CT/discography. *Spine* 1987;12:295–298.
47. Walsh T, Weinstein JN, Spratt KF. Lumbar discography in normal subjects. *J Bone Joint Surg Inc* 1990;72A:1081–1088.
48. Weatherley CR, Prickett CF, O'Brien JP. Discogenic pain persisting despite solid posterior fusion. *J Bone Joint Surg (Br)* 1986;68:142–143.
49. Wilkinson HA, Schuman N. Intradiscal corticosteroids in the treatment of lumbar and cervical disc problems. *Spine* 1980;5:385–389.
50. Yu SW, Haughton VM, Sether LA, Wagner M. Comparison of MR and discography in detecting radial tears of the annulus: A post mortem study. *AJNR* 1989;10:1077–1081.

IMAGE-GUIDED PAIN MANAGEMENT
edited by P. S. Thomas.
Lippincott–Raven Publishers, Philadelphia © 1997

20

Spinal Cord Stimulation: Stage I

P. Sebastian Thomas and Christi Barber

*Department of Anesthesiology, SUNY Health Science Center at Syracuse,
Syracuse, New York 13210*

The early 1960s saw the beginning of a new treatment for some chronic pain syndromes, known as *Dorsal Column Stimulation* (DCS). Implantation of the first system into the dorsal columns was accomplished in 1967 by C. Norman Shealy, a neurosurgeon. Although the exact physiological method of action is not clear, the most probable explanation can be found in the Melzack and Wall Gate Control Theory of pain inhibition. The theory states the nociceptive impulses to the spinal cord are blocked by low-voltage stimulation of the large diameter nerve fibers.

Implantation of the then flat, wide leads with closely spaced electrodes was performed through laminotomy by either neuro- or orthopedic surgeons. Although the system was frequently definitive in the treatment of appropriate chronic pain syndromes, it lost favor among practitioners due to drawbacks inherent in the system. The laminotomy in and of itself was invasive and could become a new cause of chronic pain. The leads could cause neurological deficits. The lead was difficult to place effectively because the patient was under general anesthesia. In time, the lead could migrate both laterally and longitudinally and eventually deprive the patient of the appropriate areas of stimulation.

In the early 1970s, new leads were developed that could be percutaneously inserted. This allowed nonsurgical practitioners such as anesthesiologists to become involved with the system and negated most of the previously mentioned complications and drawbacks. Laminotomy need not be performed and, therefore, the patient could remain awake and participate in identification of the maximum area of stimulation. Although the lead can still migrate longitudinally, the addition of multiple, varyingly spaced electrodes allows wide variation in the pattern of stimulation. Use of fluoroscopy further enhances the practitioners' ability to fine tune placement of the lead. The advancements have allowed the choice of *Spinal Cord Stimulation* (SCS) as a chronic pain treatment modality to grow in popularity.

Chronic pain is managed along a classic continuum beginning with the most conservative treatment such as medications, through physical therapy and blocks, and finally into the invasive procedures. SCS is at the end of this continuum next to implantation of morphine infusion pumps and just prior to neuroablation. SCS presents as viable therapy for nonoperative, intractable pain syndromes because, although it is invasive, it is both nondestructive and easily reversible. It has the added advantage of the trial phase known as Stage I which allows the patient and practitioner the ability to test it in a real situation.

INDICATIONS

Neuropathic pain is the primary indication for consideration of SCS. Neuropathic pain is usually resistant to narcotics. The pain syndromes most commonly and effectively treated are (1,2,4–14):

1. Sympathetically mediated pain
   a. Reflex Sympathetic Dystrophy (RSD)
   b. Causalgia
2. Post laminectomy/Failed Back Syndrome
3. Cervical or lumbosacral radiculitis
4. Phantom limb/post amputation neuralgia
5. Peripheral vascular disease
6. Post-herpetic neuralgia
7. Ischemic pain
8. Arachnoiditis

SELECTION CRITERIA

The selection criteria followed at the Pain Treatment Service, Department of Anesthesiology, SUNY Health Science Center are:

1. The patient must have chronic intractable pain
2. Must have defined pathology, preferably of a dermatomal nature
3. Must have exhausted all other appropriate conservative treatment modalities such as medication, blocks, and TENS
4. Must not be exhibiting uncontrolled drug-seeking behavior
5. Must have undergone a thorough psychiatric evaluation which examines the patient's ability to cope with an implanted device as well as their motivation and understanding of the procedure
6. Following extensive patient and family education, must demonstrate understanding of their role and a willingness to participate in the implantation procedure and the recovery/rehabilitation phases
7. Must have a clearly defined support system and appropriate psychological and physical environment for post-operative recovery

CONTRAINDICATIONS

1. Bleeding diathesis
2. Infection in the area of implantation
3. The antithesis of the above-listed inclusion criteria.

EQUIPMENT SELECTION AND LEAD PLACEMENT

Two major companies, Medtronic and Neuromed produce and service SCS systems. There are differences in the systems which need to be considered when selecting the system and the leads for the individual patient. Both companies now produce systems that are driven by either external or internal power sources. The choice between these requires input from the patient as the external source requires the wearing of an external antennae and a transmitter. The external system does have the advantage of using a 9-volt rechargeable battery which obviously does not require surgery for replacement. The internal system is favored for body image and use in water. Obviously, the selection of the type of electrodes depends on the patient and the physician.

Selection and placement of the lead is also made at this time. The various configurations of the electrodes, as well as number of electrodes and the use of single or multiple leads are based on the specific pain distribution. The schematic representation of the actual relation of the nerve root to the affected dermatome is illustrated in the *Management of Pain* by Bonica (3).

This placement may be modified during the surgery, based on patient response. At this time, the patient should also make known their preference for placement of the battery or receiver.

METHOD

Following appropriate pre-operative protocols, patients are admitted to the hospital on the operative day and prepared for routine minor surgery. The majority of patients undergo this procedure with only local anesthesia and routine nursing monitoring, but some may necessitate the use of MAC. An IV is inserted and a broad spectrum antibiotic is infused. The IV is maintained at KVO for immediate access if any untoward action should occur and for administration of sedation or pain medication if the need arises. The patient is placed prone on an appropriately padded OR table. Lumbar lead placement requires extra pillows under the abdomen to assist with proper flexion. Cervical placement can be aided with the use of a foam "doughnut" under the forehead to keep the spine aligned and flexed. The operative area is unsterily draped off with 3M drapes. The area is then prepped with Betadine scrub and solution or Hibiclens as allergies warrant and then draped in routine fashion. At this juncture, fluoroscopy via C-arm is employed to identify the correct lumbar or thoracic level. Local anesthetic is administered and a small midline incision is made. The components of the various SCS systems always include a 15-gauge Tuohy needle, which is now employed to enter at a shallow angle the epidural space using LOR technique. A flexible guidewire is inserted into the space and advanced to the previously determined level. The guidewire is removed and the lead is inserted. Fluoroscopy is used at this time to track the lead as it proceeds into the epidural space. Both AP and lateral views are required to determine posterior versus anterior placement (Figs. 1 and 2). The fluoroscopy is also needed to confirm placement of a single lead at or near midline and L/R placement of dual leads (Figs. 3 and 4). At this time, the lead is connected to the sterile test cable and stimulator box. As the patient is awake, they are able to describe the type of sensation and the precise location of the stimulation. Placement of the lead is modified based on this input. At this time, it is necessary to obtain greater than 20% relief. Permanent films are stored to record this optimal placement. The cable and screener are now removed. Blunt dissection is completed within the midline incision to allow anchoring of the lead. The Tuohy needle is removed while under fluoroscopy and lead placement is compared with the stored image. If necessary the cable and screener may be reconnected and retested. The anchor is slipped over the lead and sutured to the ligament with 2-0 silk ligature. The area lateral to the midline incision is anesthetized with local anesthetic and the tunneling tool and sheath are employed to pass the extension set from the midline incision to the lateral percutaneous stab wound site. The extension is attached to the permanent lead by carefully tightening the set screws. A silicone boot is secured over this connection with a 2-0 silk tie. Further dissection is employed to create a small pocket for containment of this connection assembly. The lead and connector are carefully placed into the pocket ensuring some slack and no sharp kinks in the lead or extension. The midline

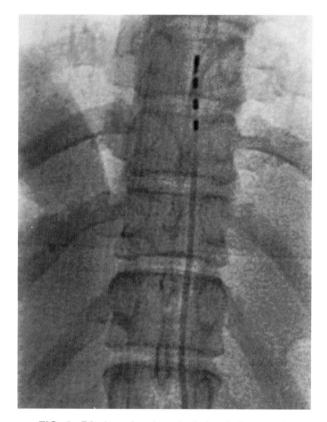

FIG. 1. PA view showing single lead placement.

incision is inspected for final hemostasis, irrigated with antibiotic solution, and closed in a routine manner. The test cable is reconnected to the end of the exposed extension and both the incision and exit stab wound are dressed with antibiotic ointment, 4 x 4's and Tegaderm. The patient is then transferred to either post-operative recovery or directly to the nursing unit bed where they remain on bedrest overnight. They are given adequate pain medication and a soft cervical collar if a cervical lead was placed. Trial stimulation may begin at this point or in the morning when they are more comfortable, if they so choose.

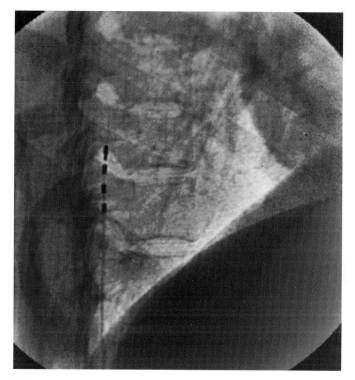

FIG. 2. Lateral view showing posterior placement of single lead.

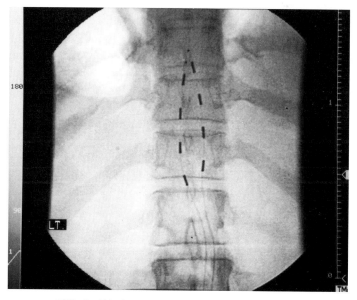

FIG. 3. PA view showing dual lead placement.

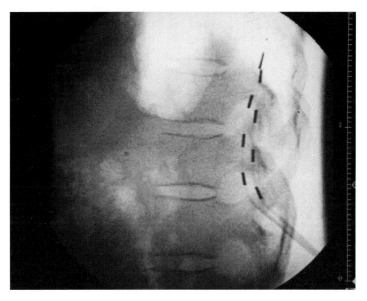

FIG. 4. Lateral view showing posterior placement of dual lead.

TESTING PROCEDURE

Patients are asked to try to recreate their pre-implant pain patterns during their 2-day hospital stay. Some patients prefer to return home during this time and if it is logistically feasible, it is a viable option. The company representative and pain management staff work with the patient to teach them how to use the equipment and to try all the various options to test their pain control.

Patients are asked to rate their pain on both a VAS and as a percentage of improvement. The protocol used in our institution requires a 50% improvement in their pain before we finalize plans for Stage II implantation of the power source. Patients and family are encouraged to participate fully in this decision.

COMPLICATIONS

Complications may occur and cause practitioners to abort Stage II or may occur at a later time and require intervention and or removal of the SCS. The most common complications include but are not necessarily limited to:

1. Infection
2. Dural tap
3. Hematoma
4. Nerve damage

REFERENCES

1. Barolat G, et al. Epidural spinal cord stimulation in the management of reflex sympathetic dystrophy. *Stereotact Functional Neurosurg* 1989;53: 29–39.
2. Bedder M. The anesthesiologist's role in neuroaugmentative pain control techniques: Spinal cord stimulation and neuraxial narcotics. *Profess Anesthesiol* 1990;4:226–235.
3. Bonica JJ. *The management of pain, Vol 1*. Lea and Febiger, Malvern, Pennsylvania; 1990.
4. Broseta J. Spinal cord stimulation in peripheral arterial disease. *J Neurosurg* 1986;64:71–80.
5. Burton CV. Clinical significance of lumbosacral adhesive arachnoiditis. *Curr Ther Neurol Surg* 1989;2:289–290.
6. DeVulder J, et al. Spinal cord stimulation in chronic pain therapy. *Clin J Pain* 1990;6:51–56.
7. Graber J, Lifson A. The use of SCS for severe limb threatening ischemia; a preliminary report. *Annal Vascular Surg* 1987;5:578–582.
8. Ray CD. The implantation of spinal cord stimulators for relief of chronic and severe pain. In: *Lumbar spine surgery*. Williams & Wilkins, Baltimore, Maryland; 1988:350–370.
9. Jacobs M, et al. Foot salvage and improvement of microvascular blood flow as a result of epidural spinal electrical stimulation. *J Vascular Surg* 1990;12:354–360.
10. Kumar K, et al. Treatment of chronic pain by epidural spinal cord stimulation: A 10-year experience. *J Neurosurg* 1991:402–407.
11. Lazorthes Y, Verdie JC. Technical evolution and long term results of chronic spinal cord stimulation. *Neurostimulation: An overview*. Futura, Mt. Kisco, New York; 1985:67–86.
12. LaPorte C, Siegfried J. Lumbosacral spinal fibrosis (spinal arachnoiditis). *Spine* 1983;8:593–603.
13. North R, et al. Failed back surgery syndrome: 5-year follow-up after spinal cord stimulation implantation. *Neurosurg* 1991;28:692–699.
14. Robaina FJ, et al. Spinal cord stimulation for relief of chronic pain in vasospastic disorders of the upper limbs. *Neurosurg* 1989;24:63–67.

IMAGE-GUIDED PAIN MANAGEMENT
edited by P. S. Thomas.
Lippincott–Raven Publishers, Philadelphia © 1997

21

Spinal Cord Stimulation: Stage II Implantation

James W. Holsapple

Department of Neurological Surgery, SUNY Health Science Center at Syracuse, Syracuse, New York 13210

SELECTION OF PATIENTS FOR STAGE II IMPLANTATION

After successful Stage I implantation of a dorsal column stimulator, the patients are allowed 2 to 3 days to ad-lib electrode stimulation with a bedside pulse generator. In this way, patients are able to ascertain whether or not the electrode system has been properly placed and generates useful paresthesias. The night before Stage II implantation, patients are interviewed by a fresh objective team of physicians and asked to rate the effectiveness of the system. If patients feel that the stimulated paresthesias sufficiently mask the effective body part, Stage II procedure is indicated.

Because Stage II requires placing permanent electrode leads beneath the skin and the placement of a pulse generator in the flank or abdominal wall, the patient's abdomen and chest are carefully evaluated prior to Stage I. If extensive abdominal surgery or chest-wall injury makes subcutaneous placement of electrode and pulse-generator placement impossible, Stage I is not pursued. If, on the other hand, this is not the case or only minor prior abdominal surgery had been performed, a judicious choice for final position can be made.

OPERATIVE TECHNIQUE/GENERATOR
PLACEMENT

The patient is taken to the operating room and general anesthesia is administered. In some institutions, Stage II implantation is performed with a local anesthetic. It has been our experience, however, that extensive subcutaneous tracking and pocket construction is difficult with local anesthetics.

Following induction of general anesthesia, the patient is placed in a lateral decubitus position with both arms extended and raised above shoulder length. An axillary roll is usually placed beneath the downside axilla. The abdomen, flank, and back are then shaved. The electrode lead is then disconnected from the external-pulse generator and cut at skin level with a pair of clean scissors with slight traction on the electrode wires to allow retraction of relatively clean electrode material into the subcutaneous tissue. All other dressings over the prior Stage I incision site are removed. Previously placed nylon sutures are not removed. The entire field is then prepped with Betadine or alcohol and draped.

The midline Stage I incision is then reopened and all stitches removed. The proximal electrode connection is then withdrawn from the incision and disconnected from the temporary remaining distal electrode leads. These are then removed completely from the operative field and the incision in the proximal remaining ends of the electrode leads irrigated with high concentration Bacitracin solution. Depending on a prior choice of generator type (battery, induction coil) and the patient's preferred site, an incision is then made in either the upper quadrant of the abdomen or along the flank at least 2 to 3 finger breadths below the costal margin. The incision is usually 2 to 3 cm in length. The incision is made with a scalpel and a retractor placed in the wound. Subcutaneous bleeders are coagulated and using scissors, a pocket beneath the surface large enough to accommodate a pulse generator, or induction coil is fashioned. Using a Salmon passer, a track in the subcutaneous fat is then made which connects this incision site with the previously reopened Stage I incision. If the track is short, the electrode leads may be placed within the passer itself and pulled proximal to distal and into the abdominal pocket. Longer tracks may require the placement of large silk tie within the track that can then be used to gently pull the electrode leads from Stage I incision site to generator pocket incision site. Once this is done (Fig. 1), both incision sites are then vigorously irrigated with Bacitracin solution.

Electrode leads are fastened to a battery pack or induction coil system and all connections checked by two operators for tightness and security. The generator is then placed in the subcutaneous pocket (Fig. 2) and both incisions closed. The dermis is closed with an inverted 3-0 Vicryl stitch. The skin is

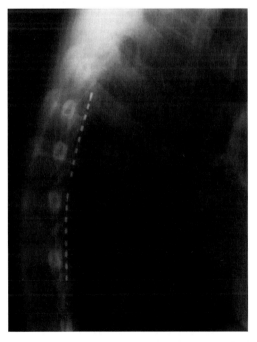

FIG. 1. Lateral view showing final lead placement before battery insertion.

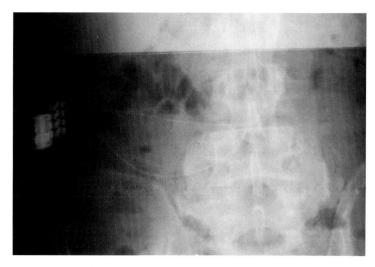

FIG. 2. PA view showing leads connected to the implanted battery.

closed with a running lock 3-0 nylon stitch. Both incisions are covered with Bacitracin ointment and dressed.

Postoperatively, the patients remain in the hospital overnight and are given 2 to 3 doses of IV antibiotics. The patients are seen 1 to 2 weeks later by the surgical staff for removal of stitches and examination of wounds.

Subject Index

Page numbers followed by *f* indicate figures; page numbers followed by *t* refer to tables.

187

ISBN 0-397-51743-2

9 780397 517435